María del Pilar Díaz Martínez

RESPIRATORY PATHOLOGIES

María del Pilar Díaz Martínez

RESPIRATORY PATHOLOGIES

Comprehensive approach from Physiotherapy

ScienciaScripts

Imprint

Any brand names and product names mentioned in this book are subject to trademark, brand or patent protection and are trademarks or registered trademarks of their respective holders. The use of brand names, product names, common names, trade names, product descriptions etc. even without a particular marking in this work is in no way to be construed to mean that such names may be regarded as unrestricted in respect of trademark and brand protection legislation and could thus be used by anyone.

Cover image: www.ingimage.com

This book is a translation from the original published under ISBN 978-613-9-40301-1.

Publisher:
Sciencia Scripts
is a trademark of
Dodo Books Indian Ocean Ltd. and OmniScriptum S.R.L publishing group

120 High Road, East Finchley, London, N2 9ED, United Kingdom
Str. Armeneasca 28/1, office 1, Chisinau MD-2012, Republic of Moldova, Europe
Printed at: see last page
ISBN: 978-620-7-75998-9

TABLE OF CONTENTS

1. <u>INTRODUCTION TO RESPIRATORY PHYSIOTHERAPY</u>

1.1. History and evolution of respiratory physiotherapy.

The history and evolution of respiratory physiotherapy is closely linked to the progress of medicine and the understanding of respiratory diseases. Over time, it has undergone significant development, from its earliest records to the sophisticated discipline it is today.

During the 19th century, the high incidence of respiratory infections and the limited availability of treatments led to the development of complementary therapies to improve the efficacy of existing treatments. Thus, in 1901, postural drainage was introduced to facilitate the elimination of secretions in patients with bronchiectasis and chronic bronchial infections, taking advantage of gravity for this purpose. With advances in the understanding of respiratory physiology, more specialized techniques for the treatment of pulmonary diseases began to emerge in Europe (1). Pioneers such as the German physician Dr. Hermann Brehmer introduced the concept of "climatic cure" for the treatment of tuberculosis, recognizing the importance of fresh air and physical exercise in the treatment of these diseases (2).

At the beginning of the 20th century, with the advent of physiotherapy as a formal discipline, especially after World War I, more systematic techniques for the treatment of respiratory pathologies were developed. Specialized clinics were established for the treatment of tuberculosis, where respiratory exercises, postural drainage and other techniques were implemented to improve pulmonary function. Throughout the 20th century, specific respiratory physiotherapy techniques were developed and refined, such as mechanical ventilation, postural drainage, percussion and vibration, among others. These techniques became mainstays in the treatment of a variety of respiratory diseases, from chronic bronchitis to acute respiratory distress syndrome (ARDS) (3). In the 1940s, the Anglo-Saxon school, prominent in Europe, promoted techniques centered on gravity, shock waves and forced expiration (F.E.T.). These practices were known as Conventional or Standard Respiratory Physiotherapy Techniques. On the other hand, the French school advocated secretion drainage techniques, in contrast to those based on airflow variations of the Anglo-Saxon school. During the 1950s, the focus on postural drainage and respiratory exercises acquired significant importance in the management of respiratory complications. This was because, as symptomatic improvements were observed in patients, a solid physiological basis for these therapies could be established. In 1953, the combined use of postural drainage with percussions (known as "clapping"), vibrations and bronchodilators was recorded for the first time, proving to be more effective than respiratory exercises in the treatment of post-surgical atelectasis. During a polio epidemic in Denmark, techniques such as endotracheal intubation and manual ventilation were used to keep patients breathing. At the Consensus Conference in Lyon, 1994, a model of "active" Respiratory Physiotherapy was established, based on such variations. The conclusions of this conference highlighted the efficacy of secretion drainage by controlling expiratory flow, regardless of the technique used, and underlined the widespread acceptance of physiotherapy in the treatment of bronchial hygiene (4).

In the 21st century, respiratory physiotherapy has continued to evolve with the development of more personalized and patient-centered approaches. Emphasis has been placed on the importance of pulmonary rehabilitation and physical exercise in the management of chronic respiratory diseases, as well as the crucial role of the physiotherapist in the prevention and treatment of respiratory complications in critically ill patients (5). With the advancement of medical technology, respiratory physiotherapy has undergone a revolution. Increasingly sophisticated devices and equipment have been developed, such as mechanical ventilators, inhaler spacing devices, and noninvasive ventilation systems, which have significantly improved the ability of physical therapists to treat patients with respiratory disease (6).

In 2000, international conferences on instrumental respiratory physiotherapy were held, with communications from experts who evaluated these techniques and made recommendations. Currently, the American Thoracic Society (ATS), the European Respiratory Society (ERS) and the Spanish Society of Pneumology and Thoracic Surgery (SEPAR) recommend respiratory rehabilitation for patients with chronic respiratory diseases, and the latter (SEPAR) has published a manual on Manual and Instrumental Techniques for secretion drainage, with the aim of improving knowledge of the respiratory techniques used in clinical practice (4).

1.2. Definition of respiratory physiotherapy and its importance in the treatment of pulmonary pathologies.

Respiratory physiotherapy is a specialized area within the field of physiotherapy that focuses on the diagnosis, evaluation, treatment and prevention of acute and chronic respiratory disorders. It is performed through a variety of therapeutic techniques and modalities, with the primary objective being to improve respiratory function, reduce symptoms associated with pulmonary diseases and improve the quality of life of patients affected by respiratory pathologies. To fully understand the nature and scope of respiratory physiotherapy, it is essential to explore its different aspects and how they are applied in clinical practice (3).

First, respiratory assessment plays a key role in respiratory physiotherapy. This involves a thorough diagnosis of the patient's pulmonary and respiratory function, which may include pulmonary function tests, analysis of respiratory mechanics, assessment of exercise capacity, and a detailed clinical evaluation of respiratory symptoms. This assessment provides the physical therapist with an in-depth understanding of the nature and severity of the patient's lung disease, which is essential for designing an individualized treatment plan (7).

It is important to note that respiratory physiotherapy is performed from a multidisciplinary approach in collaboration with other health professionals. This collaboration allows for comprehensive and coordinated care for patients with complex respiratory diseases, ensuring that all aspects of their care are effectively addressed. Based on the assessment findings, the physical therapist develops a customized treatment plan that addresses the patient's specific needs. This treatment plan may include a variety of techniques and modalities designed to improve respiratory function. Among these techniques are breathing exercises, which help strengthen the respiratory muscles and improve the efficiency of the respiratory system. In addition, bronchial drainage techniques, such as percussion and vibration, are used to help remove lung secretions and improve ventilation. Prevention of respiratory complications is another key aspect of respiratory physical therapy. Physical therapists work to prevent the accumulation of secretions in the lungs, improve lung expansion and strengthen respiratory muscles to reduce the risk of respiratory infections, atelectasis and other respiratory problems. In addition to the treatment of existing respiratory diseases, respiratory physiotherapy also plays an important role in pulmonary rehabilitation. Pulmonary rehabilitation programs often include supervised physical exercise, lung disease education, dyspnea management, and emotional support to help patients improve their functional capacity and quality of life (8).

In Spain, following the example of other European countries, physiotherapists are increasingly opting for specialization, reaching the highest academic degree (doctorate) and advanced levels of scientific and technical knowledge. As a result, we have highly qualified professionals to perform accurate diagnoses and treatments in respiratory physiotherapy. This fully justifies the crucial role of therapy in the management of secretion obstruction. As a conclusion, specialization in respiratory physiotherapy is distinguished both in the programs of the Degree in Physiotherapy and in postgraduate education, such as Masters, experts, specialists with defined competences recognized in the order CIN/2135/2008 and in the White Book of Physiotherapy. This knowledge provides physiotherapists specialized in the respiratory area with the ability to assess, treat and prevent complications of the respiratory system with full technical and scientific autonomy (4).

1.3. Objectives of respiratory physiotherapy.

Respiratory physiotherapy is the part of physiotherapy that, through the application of non-ionizing physical agents, evaluates the respiratory patient, establishes the therapeutic guideline and applies physiotherapeutic procedures with the aim of preventing, curing and/or stabilizing thoracopulmonary system disorders. As the concept of respiratory physiotherapy itself states, the general objective is to prevent, cure and/or stabilize patients with respiratory pathology or any other pathology that may cause respiratory complications (9).

Specific objectives include:

- Improve respiratory function.
- Prevent complications
- Permeabilize the airway of secretions. Improve pulmonary distensibility.
- Improve diaphragmatic and costal kinetics.
- Re-educate the ventilatory pattern.
- Control hyperventilation, dyspnea and muscle fatigue.
- Strengthening the respiratory musculature.
- To help in the readaptation to the effort
- Improving quality of life

2. <u>ANATOMY AND PHYSIOLOGY OF THE RESPIRATORY SYSTEM</u>

2.1. Anatomical structures of the respiratory system

The thorax acts as a protective shield for the organs related to respiration. Its bony structure is composed of the spine, ribs, sternum and scapulae (10).

The ribs articulate posteriorly with the spine and anteriorly with the sternum. The first seven ribs attach directly to the sternum, while the next three ribs fuse together and form the costal arch. The two lower ribs (11th and 12th) are known as floating ribs because they do not connect to the sternum. The space between each rib is known as the intercostal space, named after the adjacent upper rib (10).

The sternum consists of three parts: the manubrium, the body and the xiphoid appendage. Between the manubrium and the body is the sternal angle, also called the angle of Louis, which serves as an anatomical landmark. The second rib is inserted at this level, which facilitates its palpation and allows counting the ribs downward. Within the rib cage are important structures, such as the lungs and various mediastinal structures, including the heart, trachea, esophagus, lymph nodes, aorta and venae cavae (10).

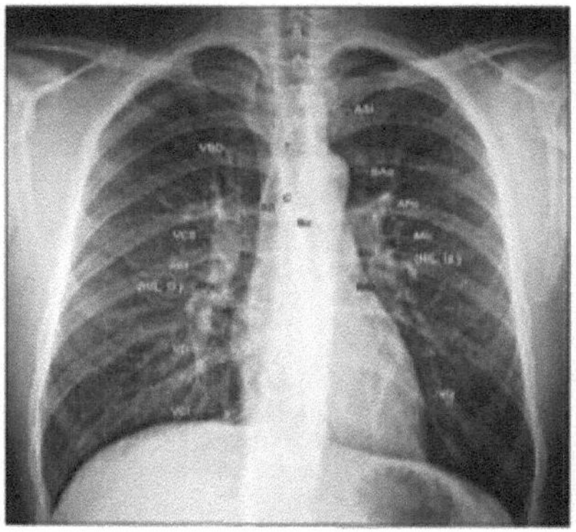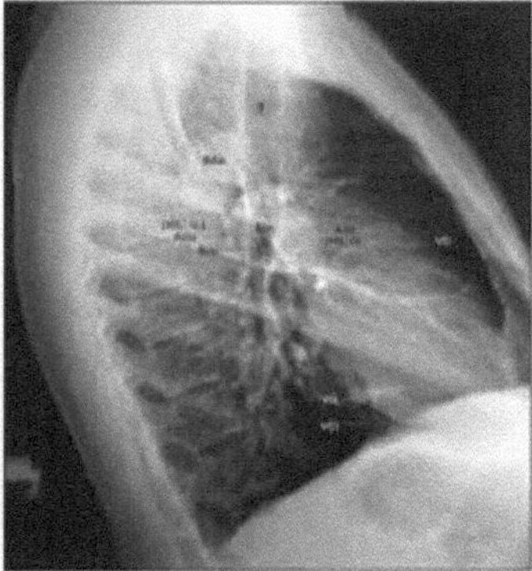

Figure 1. Simple chest radiography in anterior-postero-anterior projection and lateral radiography (10).

In addition, based on anatomical references, it is possible to draw lines and establish regions that facilitate palpation (11).

- Lines on the front:
  - The midsternal line extends from the sternal notch to the apex of the xiphoid appendage.
  - The midclavicular lines, both right and left, pass through the middle of the clavicles.
- Lines on the back:
  - The vertebral line follows the path of the spinous processes of the vertebrae.
  - The scapular lines, right and left, pass through the vertex of the scapulae.
- Lines on the side:
  - The anterior axillary line runs along the front of the axilla.
  - The median axillary line crosses the axilla at its midpoint.
  - The posterior axillary line is located at the back of the armpit.

From these lines, the following regions can be defined:

- On the front:
  - Supraclavicular region.
  - Infraclavicular region.
  - Mammary region.
  - Submammary region.
- On the back:
  - Suprascapular region.
  - Scapular region.
  - Interscapulovertebral region.
  - Infraclavicular region.

2.1.1. Oral Cavity

The oral cavity is delimited by the lips in the anterior part and the palatoglossal folds in the posterior part. At its upper limit are the hard palate and the soft palate. The floor of the oral cavity is formed by the anterior two thirds of the tongue, and in the anterior part are the teeth (10, 11).

2.1.2. Nasal Cavity

The nasal cavity extends from the nares in the anterior part to the choanae in the posterior part. This structure plays a crucial role in humidifying and warming the inhaled air. The upper part of the nasal cavity is bony, known as the bridge of the nose, composed of nasal bones, part of the maxilla and the nasal portion of the frontal bone. The floor is formed by the hard palate, which separates the nasal cavity from the mouth. The nasal septum divides the nasal cavity into two nostrils. The lateral walls contain three bony projections called turbinates, which have in their lower part the meatuses where the paranasal sinuses flow. The nostrils open to the outside through the nasal orifices and connect with the nasopharynx through the choanae. They are lined by vibrissae, which trap large particles, while smaller particles are trapped in a layer of mucus secreted by mucous cells. The olfactory mucosa, which contains the olfactory receptors, is located in the upper third of the nasal cavity (10, 11).

2.1.3. Pharynx

The pharynx is a tube that continues from the mouth and extends to the base of the skull, ending at the level of the C6 vertebra. It plays a role in swallowing and communicates with the nose, mouth and larynx. It is divided into three segments: nasopharynx, oropharynx and laryngopharynx. The nasopharynx is lined by a mucosa similar to that of the nasal cavity and has a respiratory function. The oropharynx communicates with the mouth and has a digestive function. The laryngopharynx is located behind the larynx (10, 11).

2.1.4. Larynx

The larynx is responsible for the production of sounds with the help of the vocal cords. It is located between the laryngopharynx and the trachea and consists of nine cartilages. The intrinsic muscles of the larynx control the movement of the glottis and tighten the vocal cords, while the extrinsic muscles are involved in swallowing (10, 11).

2.1.5. The Trachea

The trachea is a structure that continues from the larynx to the carina, approximately at the level of the sixth dorsal vertebra. It is a fibrocartilaginous duct about 13 cm long, with its upper half in the neck and the lower half in the thorax, which facilitates the passage of air to the lungs. It maintains its rigid shape thanks to a series of C-shaped tracheal cartilages, joined by ligaments and completed later by a membrane that allows the esophagus to adapt to it during swallowing. These cartilages, being linked by elastic fibers, allow the trachea to expand and contract. The trachea is susceptible to respiratory infections, and its cleanliness depends on the proper functioning of the cilia. It descends in front of the esophagus and gradually narrows as it descends toward the carina, where it bifurcates into the right and left main bronchi (10, 11).

2.1.6. The Bronchi

The right main bronchus is wider, vertical and shorter than the left, and is divided into three segmental bronchi: superior, middle and inferior. It continues from the trachea at a wider angle than the left bronchus. The left bronchus runs inferolaterally, passes under the arch of the aorta and anterior to the aorta and esophagus before entering the pulmonary hilum, and has two segmental bronchi: superior and inferior. The upper bronchus is considered to be further divided into superior and inferior or lingula. Each segmental or lobar bronchus supplies one lobe of the lung. Up to 23 generations of branch bronchi have been described in the lungs. The segmental bronchi divide into smaller caliber bronchioles, and after the third generation, they lose their cartilage and are renamed bronchioles. Beyond the tertiary segmental bronchioles, there are generations of ramifications called conduction bronchioles, which only conduct air. These bronchioles decrease in caliber until they become terminal bronchioles, which are the smallest part of the airway without alveoli. Each terminal bronchiole gives rise to several generations of respiratory bronchioles, which are characterized by an increasing number of alveoli (10, 11).

2.1.7. The Alveoli

The functional unit of the lung, also known as the acinus, is the terminal respiratory unit formed by the respiratory bronchioles, alveolar ducts, alveolar sacs and alveoli, where gas exchange occurs. The pulmonary alveoli are small sacs formed by a very thin layer of cells, surrounded by pulmonary blood capillaries. This thin layer allows the diffusion of oxygen and carbon dioxide. With each bifurcation of the bronchial tree, the total cross-sectional area of the ducts increases, thus decreasing the overall resistance of the airway, as its total area increases by addition (10, 11).

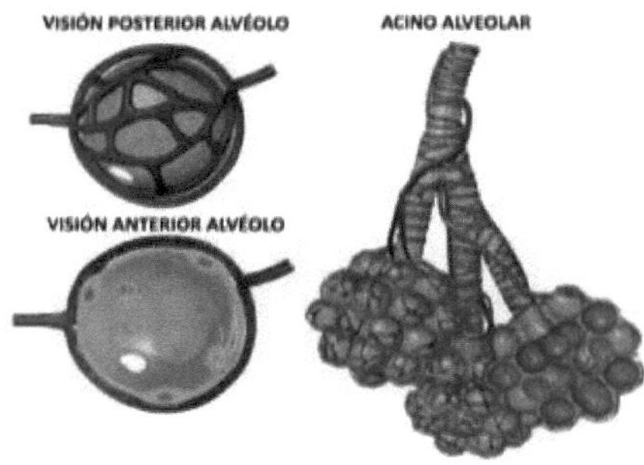

Figure 2. Representation of the pulmonary acinus and alveolus (12).

2.1.8. The Lungs

The lungs are separated by the mediastinum and consist of apex, base, lobes, faces and borders. The costal face of the lung is convex and is in contact with the costal pleura, while the mediastinal face is concave due to its relationship with the middle mediastinum and contains the hilum. The larger and heavier right lung has two fissures dividing it into three lobes, while the left lung has a single fissure and is divided into two lobes. Each lung is lined by a serous pleural sac formed by the visceral pleura and the parietal pleura, with a pleural cavity between them containing serous pleural fluid, which lubricates the pleural surfaces to facilitate breathing. The costodiaphragmatic and costomediastinal sinuses are formed between the diaphragmatic and costal, and mediastinal and costal pleurae, respectively (10, 11).

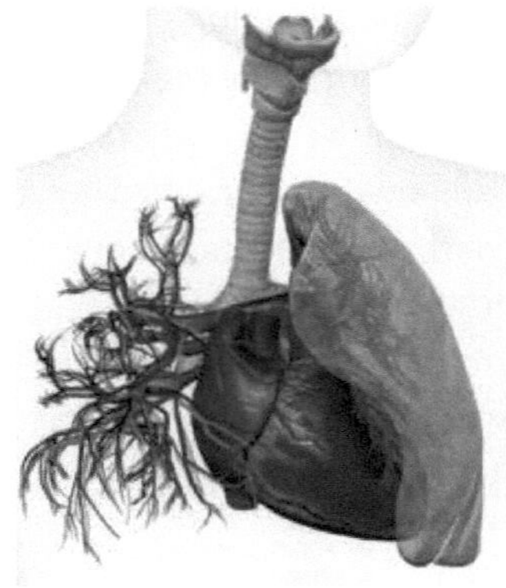

Figure 3. Representation of lungs, heart and trachea (12).

2.2. Ventilatory mechanics and pulmonary ventilation

2.2.1. Ventilatory mechanics.

In physiology, the concept of respiration is mainly focused on what is known as "external respiration". However, true respiration occurs at the cellular level, where cells use oxygen along with organic molecules to generate carbon dioxide, water and adenosine triphosphate, in a process called cellular respiration. External respiration, on the other hand, involves the exchange of gases between the body's cells and the environment through four stages (13):

- Pulmonary Ventilation: The process of intake (inspiration or inhalation) and output (expiration or exhalation) of air from the lungs. This process, active in nature, is regulated by respiratory mechanics. Ventilation corresponds to a basically mechanical phenomenon, in which the alveolar air is renewed cyclically. Three main components are involved in this process:
  - Airways: ducts that communicate the external environment with the exchange surface.
  - Thorax: protects the lung and is the engine of ventilation.
  - Lung: surface of gas exchange between air and blood.

- External gas exchange: Consists of the passive diffusion of oxygen and carbon dioxide between the alveolar air and the blood in the pulmonary capillaries.
- Gas Transport: This active process involves the transport of oxygen and carbon dioxide through the blood circulation.
- Tissue Gas Exchange: Refers to the transfer of oxygen and carbon dioxide between blood capillaries and cells, also by passive diffusion.

To carry out this respiratory process, the coordination of two main systems is required: the respiratory system, responsible for ventilation and gas exchange, and the cardiovascular system, responsible for blood perfusion in the areas of gas exchange. The respiratory system is divided into two main zones: the conduction zone and the respiratory zone. The conduction zone comprises the upper and lower airways, including the nose, mouth, pharynx, larynx, trachea, bronchi and bronchioles. Its main function is to conduct air into the respiratory zone and to perform air humidification, heating and filtration functions. On the other hand, the respiratory zone is formed by the respiratory bronchioles and alveoli, where external gas exchange takes place (13).

In relation to the characteristics and mechanical function of the respiratory system, we can describe the following fundamental pillars (9):

- Compliance or compliance, which indicates the ease with which the lungs expand during inspiration, refers to the ability of the lungs and airways to expand and contract in response to pressure changes. High distensibility indicates that the lungs can expand easily with minimal pressure changes, which facilitates lung ventilation. Distensibility decreases in conditions such as emphysema and the lungs lose their elasticity.
- Elasticity is related to the capacity of the lungs to return to their initial size after inspiration.
- Surface tension refers to the force generated on the surface of the alveoli due to the attraction between the liquid molecules on the surface. This tension tends to collapse the alveoli, making it difficult for them to expand during inspiration. To counteract this force, the

lungs produce a pulmonary surfactant, a substance that reduces surface tension and prevents alveolar collapse.

- Airway resistance refers to the opposition to airflow through the airways. To measure this resistance, it is necessary to know the pressure difference between the alveolus and the mouth, as well as the airflow. Resistance varies in different parts of the airways, being higher in the larynx, pharynx and bronchi larger than 2 mm in diameter, and lower in bronchi smaller than 2 mm. Importantly, airway resistance changes inversely proportional to lung volume. This is because the traction of the elastic lung tissue on the airway walls changes its caliber, which also results in differences in resistance between quiet and forced breathing. Increased airway resistance can hinder lung ventilation and contribute to dyspnea.

- Airway flow refers to the speed with which air moves during inspiration and expiration. Flow can be laminar (smooth and orderly flow), transitional (intermediate) or turbulent (fast and disorderly) (14). Flows are directly related to volumes. Both elements are used as a clinical tool mainly for the evaluation and monitoring of chronic diseases by generating a curve that relates them and determines the flows at 75, 50 and 25% of vital capacity (13).

Type of flow	Site	Air flow	Driving pressure	Representation
LAMINATE	Small airways	Small (low lung volumes)	Proportional to gas viscosity	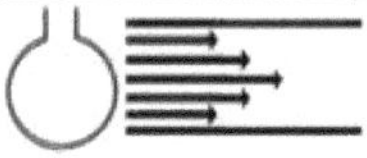
TRANSITIONAL	Branching and narrowing points	Media	Proportional to the density and viscosity of the gas	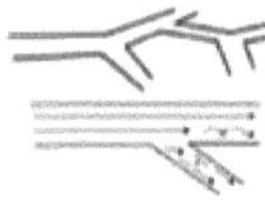
TURBULENT	Trachea and large airways	Large (large lung volumes)	Proportional to the square of the current. Depends	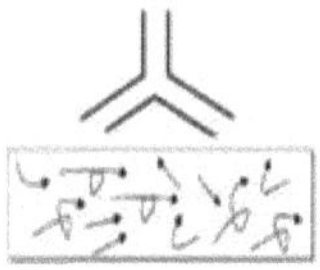

	on the density of the gas

Table 1. Summary of flow types, site of occurrence and representation.

- Rohler's equation, which describes the relationship between ventilation, elasticity and duct resistance in the respiratory system. It states that ventilation is equal to the product of elasticity and flow divided by resistance: V = E × Flow / R. This equation is important for understanding how factors such as distensibility and resistance affect pulmonary ventilation (9).
- Strength affects the capacity for muscle contraction and the tension generated. These properties are fundamental to understand the functioning and respiratory dynamics of the human body (9):
  - Starling's law applies to smooth muscle, including smooth muscle present in the airways. It states that the force of muscle contraction is directly proportional to its initial length before contraction. In the context of the airway, this means that the force of smooth muscle contraction is related to its length before contraction, which affects airway resistance and diameter.
  - Laplace's law: Laplace's law refers to the relationship between pressure, radius and surface tension in a spherical or cylindrical structure. In the pulmonary context, this law states that the pressure in the alveoli is directly proportional to the surface tension and radius of the alveoli, and inversely proportional to the thickness of the alveoli wall. This law is important for understanding how alveolar stability is maintained during respiration and how surface tension and alveolar radius influence alveolar pressure.
  - According to Poiseuille's equation, airflow into or out of the lungs depends mainly on the pressure differences or pressure gradient between the inside of the lung and the outside. This relationship is inversely proportional to the resistance of the system, meaning that greater resistance hinders airflow. For

airflow to occur, the intrapulmonary pressure must change, which is achieved by changes in lung volume. According to Boyle's Law, which describes the relationship between the pressure and volume of a gas at constant temperature, a change in lung volume results in pressure differences that allow airflow due to the pressure gradient.

2.2.2. pulmonary ventilation

Pulmonary ventilation is a vital process involving the transport of air into (inspiration) and out of (expiration) the lungs. This process is carried out cyclically and automatically to maintain an optimal gas composition in the alveoli. The respiratory cycle consists of an inspiration phase, where air enters the lungs, and an expiration phase, where air leaves the lungs. During this cycle, the respiratory muscles modify the size and shape of the rib cage, resulting in changes in lung volume and thus in intrapulmonary pressure (15).

The different phases are explained below:

- Inspiration phase: The inspiratory phase involves the transfer of gas from the atmosphere into the alveoli. Under normal conditions, this action is carried out mainly by the inspiratory muscles, which can be classified into three groups: phase producers, facilitators and accessories. The diaphragm is the main producer muscle of inspiration, generating about 80% of the required effort, complemented by the contraction of the external intercostals. Boyle-Mariotte's Law explains how muscle contraction causes this air movement, as it establishes an inversely proportional relationship between the volume and pressure of a gas at constant temperature. During inspiration, muscle contraction increases intrathoracic volume, resulting in a decrease in intrapulmonary pressure with respect to the atmosphere, creating a pressure gradient that allows air to flow into the lungs. Importantly, during inspiration, the pressure is always negative relative to atmospheric pressure, and when it equals zero, the inspiratory phase concludes. The facilitatory muscles of inspiration help to keep the intrathoracic airways patent, counteracting their tendency to collapse. The accessory muscles of the inspiratory phase intervene in pathological situations or during exercise, contributing to the increase in intrathoracic volume and negative pressure, but cannot replace the function of the main muscles (14, 15).

- Expiratory phase: Once inspiration is over, the expiratory phase begins. For this phase to take place, three initial conditions must be met: the pressure gradient of the inspiratory phase must disappear, that is, the pressure inside the alveoli must be equal to the atmospheric pressure, the volume inside the lungs must be greater than the resting volume, and the muscles of inspiration must relax. Subsequently, a pressure gradient needs to be created to allow the movement of gases from the alveoli into the atmosphere, i.e., a supra-atmospheric intrathoracic pressure must be generated for exhalation to occur. Unlike inspiration, normal expiration does not involve muscles that produce the phase, although there are muscles that facilitate and complement this process. The external intercostal muscles and the diaphragm relax, which decreases the thoracic volume below its resting value. This results in an increase in intrapulmonary pressure with respect to atmospheric pressure, which favors the outflow of air. The lungs follow Hooke's Law, which states that when a force is applied to an elastic object, it stretches in proportion to the force applied. When the inspiratory muscles cease to act, the lungs return to their resting position due to this elasticity, thus creating the pressure gradient necessary for expiration. Under normal conditions, expiration is a passive process, which means that no muscular work is required to perform it. However, during expiration, facilitator muscles, such as the internal intercostal muscles, help to stabilize the rib cage. Although their absence does not have a significant impact on normal expiration. Accessory muscles are involved in forced expiration, during exercise or in pathological conditions (14, 15).

- During the rest between respiratory cycles, atmospheric and intrapulmonary pressures equalize, which stops airflow until the next respiratory cycle.

2.3. Gas exchange in the lungs

Pulmonary ventilation involves the exchange of gases in the respiratory system, where oxygen is crucial. Ventilation refers to the process of moving air in and out of the lungs. Minute ventilation is the product of respiratory rate and tidal volume, i.e., the amount of air inspired or exhaled in each breath. Alveolar ventilation begins with ambient air, which reaches the alveoli where gas exchange occurs. During this exchange, oxygen passes from the alveoli into the blood and carbon dioxide is removed from the blood into the alveoli. This process reduces the concentration of oxygen in the alveoli and increases the concentration of carbon dioxide (13).

Atmospheric pressure and the composition of gases in the atmosphere influence the amount of oxygen available for respiration. At higher altitudes, atmospheric pressure decreases, which affects oxygen availability. Populations living at high altitudes develop physiological adaptations for better oxygen uptake. The calculation of oxygen pressure is performed by considering atmospheric pressure and gas composition. After adjusting for water vapor pressure, the inspired oxygen pressure is obtained.

The relationship between ventilation and perfusion is crucial for gas exchange and regulation of oxygen and carbon dioxide levels in the blood. The distribution of ventilation and perfusion in the lungs varies according to body position and other factors. For the lung to perform its primary function of gas exchange, two essential elements are required: adequate ventilation (V) and optimal perfusion (Q). The relationship between these two parameters (V/Q) in different areas of the lung is crucial to understanding its physiological behavior. Although the concept of V/Q ratio may seem simple, it is influenced by several physical phenomena that can complicate its understanding. Ideally, a functional lung unit consists of an alveolus and the perfusing capillary, where ventilation and perfusion are optimal and equivalent. Ideally, the ventilation rate in each unit should be equal to the perfusion rate to that same unit, resulting in a V/Q ratio equal to one (13).

However, ventilation is not evenly distributed in the lungs, mainly due to the influence of gravity. In the upright position, the alveoli at the top of the lungs are more expanded than those at the bottom, resulting in greater ventilation at the lung base. In addition, variable airway resistance and distensibility also contribute to the unequal distribution of ventilation. Because the lung does not function ideally, not all units are functional. There may be well-ventilated but poorly perfused units (dead space units), poorly ventilated but well-perfused units (shunt units), and poorly ventilated and poorly perfused units (silent units). Dead space and shunt units can cause significant alterations in gas exchange, while the impact of silent units on this process is not so relevant (14, 15).

Perfusion, on the other hand, is the process by which deoxygenated blood passes through the lungs to become oxygenated. This occurs through the pulmonary circulation, where blood passes through the capillaries around the alveoli, allowing gas exchange. The oxygenated blood then leaves the lungs and returns to the heart.

The diffusion of gases through the alveolar-capillary membranes is essential for gas exchange. Fick's law describes this process, which depends on surface area, membrane thickness and other factors (15). Gas exchange takes place in the alveoli, hollow hemispherical structures that are constantly renewed and are composed of two types of cells: type I pneumocytes, which cover most of the alveolar surface, and type II pneumocytes, which synthesize pulmonary surfactant to prevent the collapse of the alveoli. From the alveolus it moves into the capillary due to the pressure difference between the alveolar oxygen pressure (PAO2) and the capillary oxygen pressure, which is equal to the mixed venous oxygen pressure. This process follows the principles of Fick's Law, Henry's Law and Graham's Law. According to Fick's Law, the rate of diffusion of a gas across a membrane is proportional to the pressure difference on each side of the membrane, the surface area of diffusion and inversely proportional to the thickness of the membrane. Under normal conditions, the pressure difference between PAO2 and venous oxygen pressure allows oxygen to diffuse from the alveolus into the capillary, while carbon dioxide moves in the opposite direction. The large exchange surface and the thin thickness of the alveolar-capillary membrane favor diffusion efficiency. However, in practice, PAO2 and arterial oxygen pressure (PaO2) are not equal due to the presence of unoxygenated blood mixing with arterialized blood, creating an anatomical short circuit that affects the partial pressure of oxygen. This is reflected in the alveolar-arterial oxygen gradient (DAaO2), which varies between 5 and 10 mmHg when breathing air with an oxygen concentration of 21% (14).

The V/Q ratio, which is the ratio of ventilation to perfusion, is essential for normal gas exchange. If ventilation is greater than perfusion, the V/Q ratio will be greater than 1, and vice versa. An imbalance in this ratio can cause disturbances in oxygen and carbon dioxide exchange. Alterations in gas exchange may result in hypoxemia, hypercapnia or a combination of both events.

- Hypoxemia is defined as a decrease in the partial pressure of oxygen in arterial blood (PaO2), and generally reflects abnormalities in gas exchange, except in cases where hypoxemia is due to a decrease in the partial pressure of inspired oxygen (PIO2), as occurs at high altitudes or when breathing a gas mixture with oxygen concentrations below 21%. There are five main causes of hypoxemia (14):
  - Hypoxemia due to decreased IOP2.
  - Hypoxemia due to hypoventilation.
  - Hypoxemia due to diffusion disorders.
  - Hypoxemia due to imbalance in the V/Q ratio.
  - Hypoxemia due to increased shunt.

These causes may derive from various physiological or pathological conditions; identification of the underlying cause of hypoxemia is crucial to determine the appropriate treatment and correct the imbalance in gas exchange.

- Hypercapnia: The effectiveness of ventilation is assessed objectively by gasimetric analysis, especially by measuring arterial carbon dioxide pressure (PaCO2), whose magnitude depends on the ratio between CO2 production (VCO2) and alveolar ventilation (VA). The relationship is expressed as PaCO2 = KVCO2 / VA, where the constant (K) has a value of 0.863. When CO2 production exceeds alveolar ventilation, PaCO2 increases, resulting in hypercapnia. This phenomenon may occur in cases of increased tissue metabolism where the ventilatory response is inadequate, or when ventilatory efforts cannot effectively remove CO2 due to excessive production. PaCO2 may also be elevated in situations where alveolar ventilation is decreased due to respiratory problems, such as bradypnea or bronchial obstruction. On the other hand, PaCO2 decreases (hypocapnia) when alveolar ventilation exceeds CO2 production. This may occur when the respiratory system must eliminate an acid load generated by metabolic acidosis. However, it can also occur in situations of hyperventilation, such as in response to hypoxemia, pain or anxiety. In addition, hypocapnia can be caused by a decrease in CO2 production, such as during anesthesia or in cases of arterial hypotension. Continuous measurement of VCO2 can be performed using a capnometer, and VA can be calculated using tidal volume (VT) and respiratory rate (RF). Determination of anatomic dead space (ADV) and ventilation "lost" in the anatomic dead space can be used to calculate VA. In clinical practice, different methods are used to assess ventilation, including semiological assessment of clinical signs of hypo- or hyperventilation, as well as gasimetric analysis, where PaCO2 is a valuable parameter to identify ventilatory disorders (14).

2.4. Transport of gases.

Gas transport is essential for maintaining normal cellular activity, and occurs through integration between the respiratory and circulatory systems. Diffusion, driven by partial pressure gradient differences and extensive exchange surfaces, is the main mechanism of gas movement in the respiratory system. Oxygen is transported primarily in two forms: dissolved in plasma and combined with hemoglobin. Although the fraction of dissolved oxygen is minor compared to the total oxygen content, it is crucial in determining hemoglobin saturation. Hemoglobin, a protein composed of globin and heme groups, acts as a transport vehicle, taking up oxygen in the pulmonary capillaries and releasing it into the tissues according to the oxygen pressure in the plasma, as shown in the hemoglobin dissociation curve. On the other hand, carbon dioxide is produced at the mitochondrial level as a product of cellular metabolism. It is transported mainly in the form of bicarbonate in plasma, as carbamino compounds with plasma proteins or as carbonic acid after reacting with water. It is also transported through the red blood cell, where it may be dissolved in the fluid inside the cell or combined with amino groups of hemoglobin, facilitating its transport from the tissues to the lungs for elimination (16).

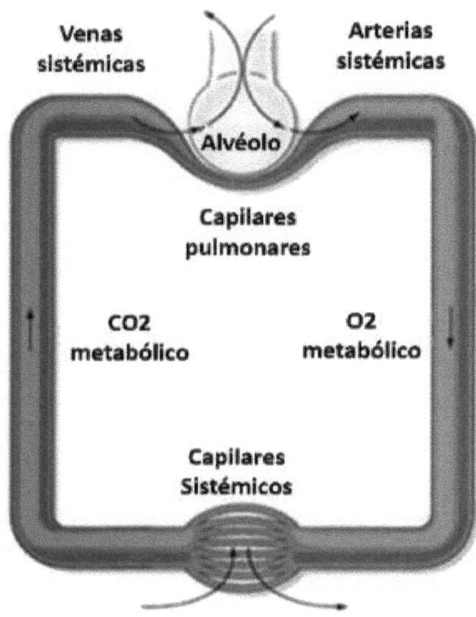

O2 and CO2 transport in arterial and venous blood (16).

2.5. Acid-base balance

Acid-base balance is essential for the proper functioning of the body, as multiple organs work together to maintain constant pH, electrical balance, osmotic balance and blood volume. The concentration of hydrogenions is crucial, as small variations can cause serious disturbances in various organs. Under normal conditions, blood pH is kept constant by the continuous production and elimination of acids and bases, carbonic acid being the most important, formed by the hydration of CO2. Buffers are solutions that limit pH fluctuations by containing a mixture of substances. The respiratory system, by means of sensors sensitive to pH changes, adjusts ventilation to increase or decrease CO2 elimination and thus maintain a constant pH. To assess acid-base balance, the Henderson-Hasselbach relationship is used, where the ratio of bicarbonate to carbonic acid reflects the behavior of the body's buffer system. The regulation of pH is strongly related to respiration, CO2 pressure and hydroelectric balance, in which the kidneys are involved. When one component of this relationship is altered, compensation occurs by modifying another component to maintain the balance. For example, if HCO3 is altered, the respiratory system adjusts PaCO2 through changes in ventilation. Although this mechanism is rapid, it has limitations, since ventilation cannot be increased indefinitely to remove CO2 or reduced excessively to retain it (16).

3. <u>METHODS OF PULMONARY FUNCTIONAL EVALUATION</u>

3.1. Functional diagnostic tests and interpretation in respiratory physiotherapy.

3.1.1. Arterial blood gases.

Arterial blood gases is an invasive technique used to evaluate pulmonary gas exchange and acid-base balance. Sampling is performed in radial, humeral or femoral arteries, and is used to diagnose and evaluate the severity and evolution of acid-base disorders. The parameters analyzed include (17):

- pH: With a normal range of 7,35-7,45. Decreased values <7.35 indicate acidosis, while increased values >7.45 indicate alkalosis.
- $PaCO_2$: With a normal range of 35-45 mmHg. Increased values >45 mmHg indicate hypercapnia, and decreased values <35 mmHg indicate hypocapnia.
- PaO_2 : With a normal range of 80-100 mmHg. Decreased values <80 mmHg indicate hypoxia.
- SaO_2 : With a normal value >95%. Decreased values <95% indicate desaturation.
- HCO_3 : With a normal range of 22-26 mEq/L. Increased values >26 mEq/L indicate increased bases, and decreased values <22 mEq/L indicate decreased bases.

Parameter		Normal	Enhanced	Decreased
pH	Acid-base balance	7,35 - 7,45	Alkalosis > 7,45	Acidosis <7,35
PaCO$_2$	Arterial partial pressure of carbon dioxide	35-45 mmHg	Hypercapnia >45	Hypocapnia <35
PaCO$_2$	Arterial oxygen pressure	80-100 mmHg	-	Hypoxia < 80
SatO$_2$	Amount of hemoglobin reduced by oxygen	>95%	-	Desaturation <95%
HCO$_3$	Bicarbonate of blood	22-26 mEq/L	Base Increase >26	Decrease in Bases <22

Summary of normal, decreased and increased parameters of the arterial range (17).

Acid-base balance and alveolar ventilation are assessed by the relationship between pH, bicarbonate concentration (HCO_3) and $PaCO_2$, related in the Henderson-Hasselbach equation. The main acid-base disturbances include (17):

- Respiratory acidosis: pH <7.35 and $PaCO_2$ >45 mmHg, caused by carbon dioxide retention.
- Respiratory alkalosis: pH >7.45 and $PaCO_2$ <35 mmHg, caused by rapid elimination of carbon dioxide.
- Metabolic acidosis: pH<7.35 and HCO_3 <22 mEq/L, caused by acid retention or loss of bicarbonate.
- Metabolic alkalosis: pH >7.45 and HCO_3 >26 mEq/L, caused by acid loss or bicarbonate retention.

A summary table of the main acid-base disturbances is shown below.

MAIN ACID-BASE DISORDERS

Acid-base balance	Causes	Compensation	pH evolution	Terminolo-gía	Symptomatology
↓ pH	PaCO2	↑ HCO3	Correction pH 7.60	Respiratory acidosis	Carbon dioxide retention. hypoventilation, caused by CNS depression (drugs or injury), asphyxia.COPD patients.
		= HCO3	pH remains acidic.		
	HCO3	↓ PaCO2	Correction pH 7.40	Metabolic acidosis	Excessive acid production (shock, Intoxications) or bicarbonate loss.
		= PaCO2	-		Compensation with hyperventilation (Kaussmaul resp.). Hyperpnea.
↑ pH	PaCO2	↓ HCO3	Correction pH 7.40	Respiratory alkalosis	Carbon dioxide elimination. Hyperventilation (anxiety, fever, hyperthermia, tachypnea). HCO3 is eliminated by urine, buffering >pH.
		= HCO3	pH remains alkaline		
	HCO3	↑ PaCO2	Correction pH 7.40	Metabolic alkalosis	Gasification of pH, loss of acids or retention of bicarbonate. Etiology Hyperemesis (loss of hydrochloric acid) or ingestion of alkalis. Slow breathing (hypoventilation), superficial, hypertonia, restlessness, twitching, confusion, apathy, convulsion, severe coma.
		= PaCO2, no change.	pH remains alkaline		

3.1.2. Pulse oximetry

Pulse oximetry is a noninvasive method that uses photoelectric methods to measure the oxygen carried by hemoglobin in blood vessels. The pulse oximeter is placed on areas of the body with good blood flow and transparency, such as the fingers, earlobe or foot. Although arterial blood gas is necessary for accurate measurement of arterial oxyhemoglobin saturation (SaO_2). Pulse oximetry provides an estimate of hemoglobin oxygen saturation, indicated as SpO_2 (saturation by arterial pulse oximetry). It is important to note that pulse oximetry provides an approximation of SpO_2 and does not provide an accurate measurement like arterial blood gases. Normal physiological saturation should be greater than 95%. Oxygen saturation values are (9):

- Normal: 95%-100% Normal: 95%-100% Normal: 95%-100% Normal: 95%-100% Normal: 95%-100% Normal: 95%-100
- Mild desaturation: 90%-94%.
- Moderate desaturation: 85%-89%.
- Severe desaturation: <84%.

The validity and reliability of conventional pulse oximeter measurements can be affected by various circumstances (18):

- Motion: Motion, especially in young children or newborns, can affect the accuracy of measurements. During movement, the length of the optics changes and can confuse the oximeter by detecting movement of venous blood as if it were arterial.
- Low perfusion: The magnitude of the signal available to the pulse oximeter depends on the perfusion of the vascular bed between the light-emitting diode and the monitor probe sensor. Low perfusion states, such as shock or hypothermia, can alter readings.
- Skin pigmentation and nail polish: Dark skin and nail polish can interfere with the oximeter's ability to interpret oxygen saturation.
- Electromagnetic interference: External electromagnetic energy, such as from CT scanners or electrocauteries, can cause interference with the oximeter reading and result in incorrect readings.

- Ambient light interference: Intense ambient light, such as phototherapy or operating room lights, can interfere with oximeter readings by altering the function of the photodetectors.
- Hemoglobin variants: The presence of carboxyhemoglobin (COHb) in the blood may overestimate arterial oxygenation values, since COHb absorbs red light in a similar manner to oxyhemoglobin. This may occur in cases of carbon monoxide (CO) poisoning or in smokers.

In addition, pulse oximetry allows continuous recording, for example, during the sleep period, in patients with suspected nocturnal hypoxemia, such as in obstructive sleep apnea syndrome (OSAS), neuromuscular diseases or COPD (19).

3.1.3. Assessment of respiratory strength.

The strength of the respiratory musculature can be assessed by measuring respiratory pressure, which includes peak inspiratory pressure (Pimax) and peak expiratory pressure (Pemax). These measurements are made using a manometer or electronic device and are expressed in centimeters of water (cmH2O). Here is a description of how the assessment is performed (20):

- Peak inspiratory pressure (Pimax): It can be measured by mouth or nose.
    - For measurement by mouth, the patient sits with a straight back in a quiet place. He/she should occlude the nose with nasal forceps. He performs an expiration up to the residual volume (RV) and then a maximal inspiration. Inspiratory effort is maintained for 3-5 seconds. At least six maneuvers are performed, with a one-minute rest between each maneuver. The three best and most reproducible maneuvers are selected. A Pimax > 75-80 cmH2O in men and > 50 cmH2O in women is considered normal.
    - For the Sniff test, 10 Sniff maneuvers are performed from the functional residual capacity (FRC) at 30-second intervals. The highest value is selected. A value above 70 cmH2O in men and > 60 cmH2O in women is considered normal.

- Peak expiratory pressure (Pemax): It is measured similarly to Pimax, but the patient performs a maximal inspiration up to total lung capacity (TLC) and then a maximal expiration. Effort is maintained for 3-5 seconds. The three best and most reproducible are selected. A Pemax > 100 cmH2O in men and > 80 cmH2O in women is considered normal.

It is important to keep in mind that reference values may vary according to the population and it is recommended to establish specific reference values for each laboratory.

3.1.4. Spirometry.

Since the introduction of the forced spirometry regulations by the Spanish Society of Pneumology and Thoracic Surgery (SEPAR) in 1985, the practice of spirometry has become widespread throughout Spain due to its simplicity and efficacy. However, it is important to note that, after 15 years, SEPAR has decided to update the procedures again, reflecting the constant evolution in this area. The aim of this review is to set out the standards necessary to ensure the accuracy and correct interpretation of spirometry results, enabling health professionals, including pulmonologists, primary care physicians and nurses, to perform the test to uniform standards (20).

Spirometry, a mainstay in the evaluation of pulmonary function, encompasses the measurement of the lungs' capacity to handle air, being essential in the diagnosis and monitoring of respiratory conditions. Through this technique, both static and dynamic volumes are explored, and lung capacities are determined, thus contributing to the identification of obstruction, restriction or a combination of both, in addition to assessing pulmonary adaptability to effort.

Spirometry measures the amount of air that the lungs can move as a function of time, represented by volume-time and flow-volume graphs. Modern equipment is equipped with pneumotachometers that allow an instantaneous reading of the flow and a differential calculation of the volume, generating the flow-volume curve, a standardized tool worldwide. There are two types of spirometers (9):

- Volume Spirometers: They are still used as a reference for calibrations. These devices are closed and consist of one part connected to the patient's airway, sealed with water (or in more modern versions, with piston or bellows, known as dry spirometers), and another part connected to a chemograph that records the volume values. Depending on the speed, the recording allows the flow to be calculated.
- Flow Spirometers or Pneumotachographs: These devices measure flow as a function of a known resistance that generates a pressure difference between both sides of the air passage. The flow information is transmitted to an analog or digital measuring system. They can vary in design and may be turbine, piston, hot wire, ultrasonic, among others.

Despite its importance, simple spirometry does not cover the assessment of key static volumes such as total lung capacity (TLC), functional residual capacity (FRC) and residual volume (RV), for which additional techniques such as helium dilution or body plethysmography are required. Forced spirometry, using a pneumotachograph, allows measurement of forced vital capacity (FVC), forced expiratory volume in the first second (FEV1) and forced expiratory flow between 25% and 75% of FVC (FEF 25-75%) (14).

In order to perform spirometry, it is necessary to have an adequate space and equipment consisting of a receiving section and a signal interpretation section. These can be volume spirometers, which were the first to be developed and are mainly used to calibrate the equipment, or flow spirometers, which initially measure the flow from a known resistance (20).

Spirometry is used for a variety of indications in the process of diagnosing respiratory diseases and assessing lung function. Some of the specific indications include (20):

- Assess pulmonary function in the presence of symptoms, signs or abnormal laboratory data (dyspnea, cyanosis, hypoxemia).
- Measure the impact of respiratory diseases such as COPD or diffuse interstitial diseases.

- To evaluate the effect of diseases of other organs on lung function, such as connective tissue diseases or rheumatoid arthritis.
- Assess individuals at risk for respiratory disease due to factors such as smoking or exposure to inorganic dust.
- Assess preoperative risks, including pulmonary reactions.
- To assess the prognosis of respiratory diseases, such as preparation for lung transplantation.
- Assess health prior to intense physical exercise, as in high-level athletes.

We can also find some contraindications, these are relative and are usually related to the inability to perform a correct forced maximal expiratory maneuver, either due to physical or psychological limitations, or in diseases with contraindications for maneuvers that increase intrathoracic pressure. They include (20):

- Lack of collaboration or understanding to perform the maneuver.
- Recent myocardial infarction (less than 1 month).
- Retinal detachment, cataract surgery, pneumothorax, recent hemoptysis.
- Chest or abdominal pain of any cause (trauma, fractures).
- Tracheostomy.
- Mouth problems, hemiparesis, mouthpiece intolerance.
- Coughing spells.
- Urinary incontinence.
- Bronchospasm.
- Chest pain.
- Pneumothorax.
- Dizziness or syncope.

The competence of the technician performing spirometry is crucial to detect and stop the test in case of complications. Do not insist on obtaining data in case the patient presents any of these complications; instead, spirometry should be postponed for another day. If we use it for follow-up (21):

- To evaluate the effectiveness of the therapeutic intervention.
- Monitor the evolution of respiratory diseases.

- Closely monitor pulmonary function in individuals exposed to noxious agents or on medication with possible adverse pulmonary effects.

It can also be used for the evaluation of disability and incapacity for work:

- Using pulmonary function as a measure of work incapacity.
- To use pulmonary function in legal expertise.

In Public Health:

- Conduct epidemiological studies.
- Contribute to clinical research.

Before performing a spirometry test, it is important that the patient follows some recommendations and prepares adequately to ensure the validity and quality of the results obtained. Here are some of the previous recommendations and preparation steps. Before spirometry, the patient should (21):

- No smoking.
- Avoid intense physical exercise at least 30 minutes before.
- Wear clothing that does not restrict breathing maneuvers.
- Avoid large meals in the previous 2 hours.
- Avoid consumption of alcohol or caffeine in the hours before.
- It is not necessary to come on an empty stomach.
- If spirometry is diagnostic, specific intervals without bronchodilator medication should be followed prior to testing, depending on the type of medication.

It is important that the patient understands the purpose and procedure of spirometry to improve their cooperation and the quality of the results. Before the test, anthropometric measurements should be taken and relevant patient data recorded. For at least 5 minutes before the test, the patient should remain seated and relaxed while being instructed on the maneuver to be performed (21).

The following are instructions on how to perform spirometry correctly (20):

- Insert the nasal forceps and mouthpiece (non-deformable) into the mouth, making sure that the lips are well sealed around it.
- Ask the patient to perform a maximal inspiration gradually and without forcing, with a short pause when reaching total lung capacity (TLC) of less than 1 second.
- Perform a rapid forced maximal exhalation until the lungs are completely emptied to the residual volume (RV).
- If required, perform a rapid maximal inspiration with maximal effort to provide inspirrometry data.
- Repeat the instructions as necessary to obtain at least three technically satisfactory maneuvers, of which at least two are reproducible, with a maximum limit of 8 attempts.
- Verify the accuracy of the tracings and record the data obtained.

The acceptance criteria are based on ATS and ERS recommendations and are as follows (20):

- Layouts must not contain artifacts.
- It is advisable to include the tracing of the initial 0.25 seconds before exhalation to evaluate the quality of the maneuver.
- There should be no amputation at the end of expiration.
- The maneuver should be initiated by retrograde extrapolation, with an extrapolated volume of less than 5% of the forced vital capacity (FVC) or 150 ml.
- It is preferred that the exhalation lasts more than 6 seconds.
- The maneuver should end when the volume change in one second does not exceed 25 ml.
- Reproducibility criteria focus on variability in FVC and forced expiratory volume in the first second (FEV1), which should be less than 200 ml or 5% in at least two of the maneuvers.
- It is important to keep in mind that not meeting the expiratory criterion for 6 or more seconds is not sufficient reason to eliminate a maneuver, since some patients may have difficulty maintaining it. It is also common to find maneuvers with abrupt cessation or defects at the beginning of expiration.

During the performance of the test, it is common to encounter errors that can invalidate the test. These include lack of maximal effort on the part of the patient, coughing during the first second, involuntary obstructions of the mouthpiece (such as the tongue or dentures), abrupt termination of the maneuver, an irregular start to the maneuver, or a duration of less than 6 seconds. It is essential to avoid these errors in order to obtain accurate and reliable results (20).

The variables studied in spirometry are (22):

- Static volumes
  - Tidal volume (TV): The amount of air inspired or exhaled in each respiratory cycle, typically around 500 ml.
  - Inspiratory reserve volume (IRV): The maximum volume of air that can be inhaled beyond a normal inhalation, approximately 3000 ml.
  - Expiratory reserve volume (ERV): The maximum volume of air that can be exhaled after a normal exhalation, about 1100 ml.
  - Residual volume (RV): The volume of air remaining in the lungs after a maximum exhalation, approximately 1200 ml.
  - Inspiratory capacity (IC): The maximum volume of air that can be inhaled after a normal exhalation, calculated by adding the VC and VRI, about 3500 ml.
  - Functional residual capacity (FRC): the volume of gas remaining in the lungs at the end of a quiet exhalation, calculated by adding RV and ERV, approximately 2300 ml.
  - Vital capacity (VC): The maximum volume of air that can be exhaled after a maximum inhalation, calculated by adding the VRI, VC and VRE, generally between 3 and 5 liters.
  - Total lung capacity (TLC): The total volume of air in the lungs at the end of a maximal inhalation, calculated by adding CV and RV, about 5900 ml.

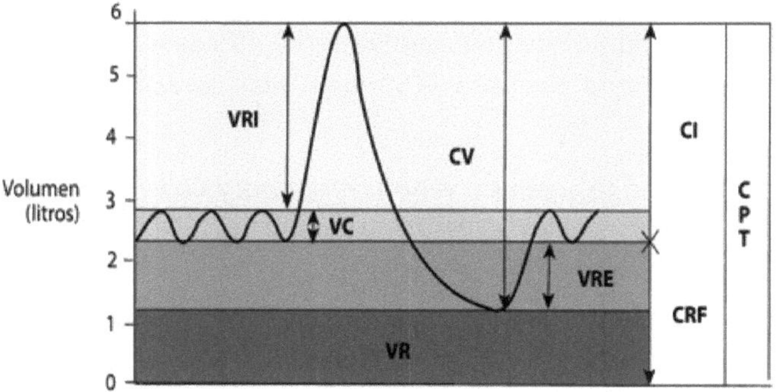

Figure 5. Representation of static lung volumes (22).

- Dynamic volumes (22):

  - Forced Vital Capacity (FVC): The maximum volume of air that can be expelled during a forced and complete exhalation from a maximum inhalation.

  - Forced Expiratory Volume in the first second (FEV1): The volume of air expelled during the first second of a complete forced exhalation from a maximal inhalation.

  - FEV1/FVC ratio: The ratio of FEV1 to FVC, usually between 0.75-0.80 (75-80%), indicating the proportion of air that can be expelled rapidly.

  - Forced Expiratory Flow 25-75% (FEF 25-75%): It is the airflow during half 50% of a forced exhalation, which evaluates the function of the small caliber airways.

  - Peak Expiratory Flow or Peak Flow (PEF or PEF): The maximum airflow during a forced exhalation, used to assess lung function, especially in asthma and COPD.

If we study the main variables, forced spirometry is based on two main variables: the Forced Vital Capacity (FVC) and the Forced Expiratory Volume in the first second (FEV1). FVC represents the maximum volume of air exhaled in a maximal effort expiratory maneuver, initiated after a maximal inspiration, and is expressed in liters. On the other hand, FEV1 corresponds to the maximum volume of air exhaled in the first second of the FVC maneuver, also expressed in liters. The FEV1/FVC ratio shows the relationship between these two variables, providing information on lung function. It should not be confused with the Tiffeneau index, which is defined as the ratio between FEV1 and vital capacity (VC) in slow spirometry (9).

In addition to volumes, various respiratory flows are considered. The mean expiratory flow (FEF25-75% or MMEF) is calculated as the flow between 25% and 75% of the forced expiratory maneuver and is expressed in liters per second. Peak expiratory flow (PEF) is obtained from the peak value on the flow-volume curve and is also expressed in liters per second. Instantaneous expiratory flows (FEFx%) refer to the flow when a certain percentage of the FVC has been exhaled, the most common being FEF25%, FEF50% and FEF75% (expressed in liters per second). These parameters are crucial for assessing lung function and can be especially useful when using simplified portable equipment (9).

Spirometry is a fundamental tool for the diagnosis, assessment of severity and follow-up of respiratory disorders. To interpret the results, it is crucial to consider both the graphical representation and the numerical values, and this interpretation must be personalized for each patient. Spirometry is considered normal when its values are above the lower limit of the confidence interval (LCI). This limit is around 80% of the theoretical value for FEV1, FVC and VC, as well as around 70% for the FEV1/FVC ratio in individuals under 65 years of age and of average height. For FEF25-75%, the LIN is around 60%. Although obstructive and restrictive ventilatory impairments are usually defined in clinical practice based on the FEV1/FVC ratio, it is recommended to use the reference equations to obtain more accurate and realistic interpretations. This allows a more complete and adequate evaluation of the pulmonary function of each patient. Obstructive ventilatory impairment is defined by a reduced FEV1/FVC ratio (below LIN). Although a criterion of 0.7 or 70% is commonly used in clinical practice, this approach may not be as accurate, resulting in false negatives in the young and false positives in the elderly (9).

Non-obstructive" ventilatory impairment is characterized by a reduced FVC with an FEV1/FVC ratio above the LIN or the mean reference value. A restrictive disorder should be suspected when the FVC is below the LIN, the FEV1/FVC ratio exceeds its LIN and the flow-volume curve presents a convex morphology. To establish the restriction grading, the ATS/ERS classification of FEV1 is also used (20).

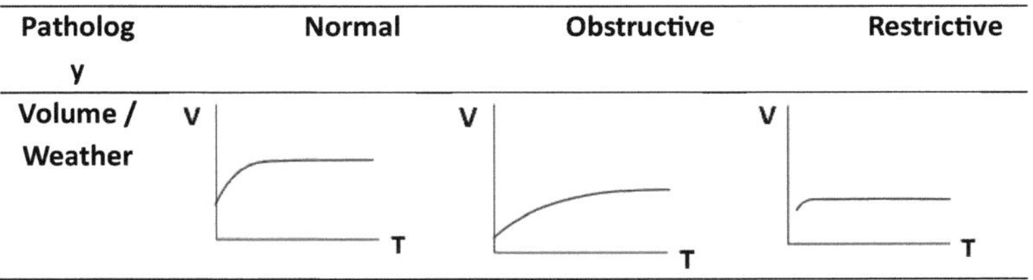

Graphical representation of the patterns according to the time/volume ratio (20).

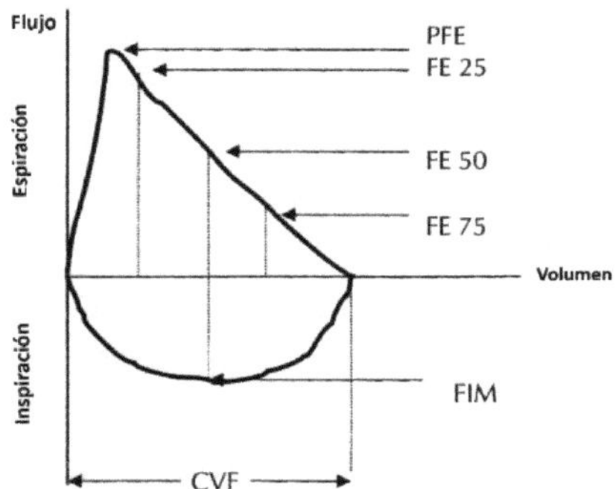

Figure 6. Graphical representation of the normal pattern of the morphology of the flow-volume curve (23).

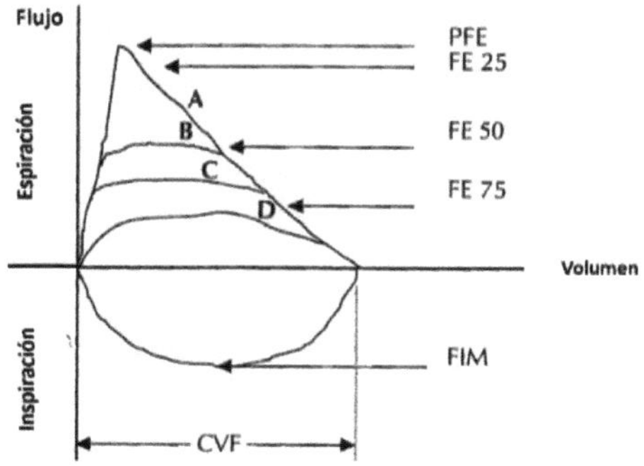

Graphic representation of alteration of the descending portion of the expiratory loop. Normal curve A, curve B, C and D represent a poorly performed procedure or a weakness of the abdominal musculature (23).

- Obstructive ventilatory disturbance.

Airflow obstruction is manifested by a disproportionate decrease in flows at low volumes, reflected in a concave shape in the flow-volume curve. Quantitatively, a proportionally greater reduction in FEF75% or FEF25-75% is observed than in FEV1. To classify obstruction, the ATS/ERS classification of FEV1 is used. Whenever an obstructive ventilatory disturbance is confirmed, a bronchodilator test (PBd) is recommended to assess whether the obstruction is reversible. This test consists of the administration of salbutamol and is evaluated if the FEV1 or FVC increases by 12% and 200 ml with respect to baseline values. Obstructive ventilatory impairment is characterized by several aspects (20):

- A reduced FEV1/FVC ratio, less than 70% (lower than LIN).
- A normal FVC, higher than 80% of reference.
- A disproportionate decrease in flow rates at low volumes, reflected in a concave shape in the flow-volume curve.
- A decrease in FEV1 or FEF25-75%. Quantitatively, a proportionally greater reduction in FEF75% or FEF25-75% or MEF 25-75% or MEF 25-75% than in FEV1 is observed.

The severity of obstructive ventilatory disorders is classified according to the FEV1 value, following the ATS/ERS recommendations (20):

FEV1 (% reference value)	Gravity
>70%	Slight
70-60%	Moderate
50-59%	Moderate - Severe
49-35%	Serious
<35%	Very Serious

Table 5. Severity classification of ventilatory alterations (20).

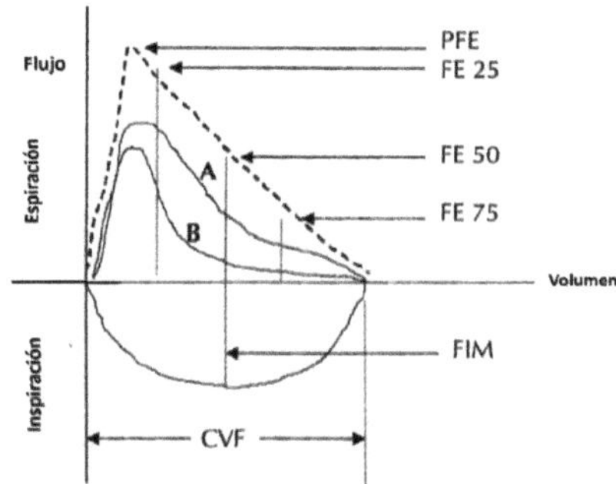

Figure 8. Flow-volume curve in obstructive disease. A and B represent obstructive pattern. However, obstruction is more severe in B because flow velocities are more diminished and the descending branch of the expiratory loop is more concave. The dotted line represents the normal flow-volume curve (23).

- Restrictive ventilatory disturbance is characterized by (20):
  - An FEV1/FVC ratio above 70% (higher than LIN) or even higher than the mean reference value.
  - A reduced FVC below the LIN.
  - In addition, a restrictive syndrome is confirmed when it is also observed:
  - A flow-volume curve of convex morphology.
  - A reduction of CPT below 80%.

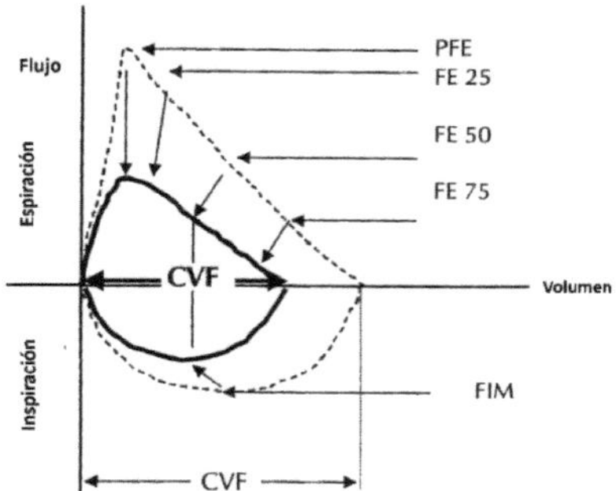

Flow-volume curve in restrictive disease (continuous line) in which FVC is lower than the expected normal (dotted line) (23).

- Mixed alteration is defined by (20):
  - A reduced FVC below the LIN.
  - An FEV1/FVC ratio below 70% (lower than LIN).
  - To distinguish whether the origin is air trapping (hyperinflation) or true restriction, CPT should be measured and the presence of restriction confirmed when FVC or VC are decreased.

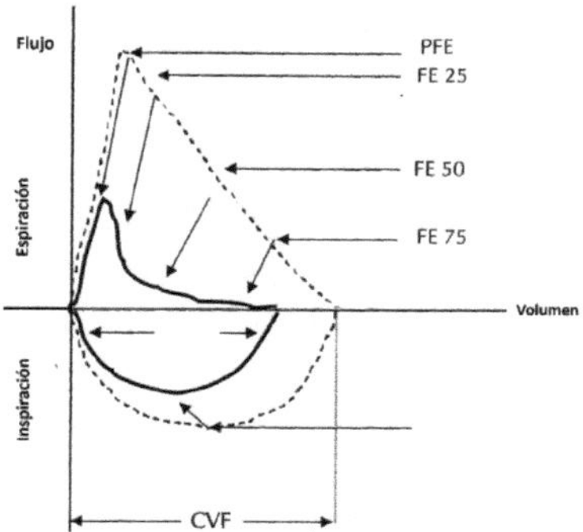

Figure 10. Flow-volume curve in mixed disease (continuous line). The dotted line represents the normal flow-volume curve (23).

SPIROMETRY			
FEV1 /FVC > 70%.		FEV1 /FVC < 70%.	
FEV1 AND FVC > 80%.	FVC < 80%.	FVC > 80	FVC < 80%.
NORMAL	**RESTRICTIVE**	**OBSTRUCTIVE**	**MIXED**

Table 6. Summary of spirometry representation

3.1.5. Auscultation:

Auscultation originated with René Laënnec, who described respiratory sounds based on a psychoacoustic analogy with the sounds of nature. In the 1970s, the use of computers to analyze these sounds led to a simpler and more scientific nomenclature, based on physical measurement parameters. Currently, the description of respiratory sounds is physicoacoustic, which allows a better understanding of lung mechanics and an objectification of physiotherapy. To understand respiratory sounds, it is important to know some simple physical parameters. Sounds are vibratory mechanical waves that are transmitted through matter. These vibrations can be periodic or aperiodic. Periodic vibrations can be simple or complex, and their analysis is based on amplitude (intensity) and period (time required for one vibration cycle), which determine the frequency (number of cycles per unit time). Complex vibrations are broken down into simple waves and Fourier analysis can be applied to examine their spectrum and determine their timbre (4).

On the other hand, aperiodic vibrations include brief and continuous pulses. The latter, like normal breath sounds, occur anarchically in time and require the use of the fast Fourier transform for their amplitude-frequency plot. All breath sounds follow a process involving an origin, transmission through a resonator and uptake by the receiver. When we perform auscultation, we are analyzing mechanical vibrations and we must pay attention mainly to the following parameters (4):

- Frequency: determines whether the sound is high-pitched (high frequency) or low-pitched (low frequency).
- Intensity or amplitude: indicates whether the sound is loud or soft. As the frequency decreases, the intensity of the sound also decreases.
- Timbre: describes the spectral composition of the sound, determining whether it is dark or light.

- Duration or time: indicates whether the sound is short or long, which may be relevant to distinguish between different types of breath sounds.

To perform an accurate and effective pulmonary auscultation, the following guidelines should be followed (4):

- Quiet Environment: Perform auscultation in a place free of ambient noises that may interfere with lung sounds.
- Quality Stethoscope: Use a good quality stethoscope to isolate sounds from the outside and improve sound transmission.
- Direct Skin Contact: Apply the stethoscope directly to the patient's skin to avoid interference caused by textile fabrics.
- Patient Position: Ideally, begin auscultation with the patient seated, as it allows for optimal bilateral comparison and homogeneous ventilation of the diaphragm. If this is not possible, you can start auscultation with the patient in supine and then in lateral decubitus to address all areas of the chest.
- Instructions to Patient: Ask the patient to take deep, regular breaths through the mouth to increase airway turbulence and facilitate sound generation and transmission.
- Auscultation Sequence: Start auscultation of the lower thorax and progress to the upper thorax. It is important to auscultate the trachea at the beginning to avoid auditory confusion. Be sure to auscultate symmetrically on both sides of the chest, except when the patient is in lateral decubitus. Auscultate at least one complete respiratory cycle at each point.
- Firm Pressure: Apply the bell of the stethoscope firmly on the skin to avoid displacements that may produce unwanted noises.
- Completion: Conclude the auscultation sequence by placing the patient in lateral decubitus on both sides. This position facilitates the transmission of lung sounds and improves ventilation and density of the lung parenchyma.

The international nomenclature described below follows the guidelines proposed by the International Lung Sounds Association (ILSA), which has been accepted by CORSA (Consortium for Standardized Respiratory Sound Analysis) and is based on the physical-acoustic properties of breath sounds. This nomenclature provides a standardized framework for the analysis of lung sounds using specialized computer software. In lung auscultation, two types of sounds are distinguished (4):

- Respiratory Sounds: They are always present and should be analyzed to detect any alteration. They are divided into (19):
  - Normal Respiratory Sounds (NR): They have a dark timbre and originate in the central and middle airways. They are filtered by the ventilated lung parenchyma and are heard mainly in the lung bases during inspiration. It has the following characteristics:
    - Low frequency.
    - Dark/severe timbre.
    - Central and middle airway origin.
    - Transmission through healthy lung parenchyma, where there is no fluid and an adequate proportion of air.
    - It can be heard throughout the chest wall, usually in the lung bases.
    - These features are useful for distinguishing between different types of breath sounds and can be used in clinical evaluation to detect possible abnormalities in the respiratory system.
  - Bronchial Respiratory Sounds (BRR): They have a clear timbre and are generated in the central and middle airways. They are heard in the chest wall and their presence may indicate consolidation of the lung parenchyma. They have the following characteristics:
    - High frequency.
    - Clear/sharp timbre.
    - Central and middle airway origin.
    - Transmission through healthy lung parenchyma.
    - It can be heard in the lung apices of a healthy adult person.
    - It is important to note that bronchial breath sounds in the lung apices are not pathologic due to the smaller amount of lung parenchyma in this area, resulting in less air and noise filtration. However, if it is found anywhere else in the

thoracic region other than the apices, it may indicate pathology.

- Tracheal Respiratory Noise (TRN): Similar to TRN, but originates in the trachea. It is important to auscultate it in adults. They have the following characteristics:
  - High frequency.
  - Clear/sharp timbre.
  - Origin in structures such as pharynx, larynx, trachea and first bronchial generation.
  - Transmission without filtration through the pulmonary parenchyma.
  - It can be perceived on both sides of the trachea.

- Adventitious sounds: These are pathological sounds that are added to normal respiratory sounds. They are divided into (19):
  - Crackles: Correspond to pulsed aperiodic vibrations and may indicate pathological bronchial secretions or sudden opening of an airway. They are classified according to the frequency and the phase of the respiratory cycle in which they occur.
    - Fine base crackles (BF):
      - They appear at the onset of inspiration.
      - They indicate the presence of secretions in the nearby airways.
      - They are audible without the use of a stethoscope.
    - Thin-middle crunches (MF):
      - They appear in the middle of inspiration.
      - They indicate the presence of secretions in the middle airway.
    - Fine apex crackles (AF):
      - They appear at the end of inspiration or at the beginning of expiration.
      - They indicate the presence of secretions in the distal pathway.
    - The genesis of these sounds can be attributed to two hypotheses:

- - -
  - Sudden opening of a previously closed airway: This type of crackles occurs in the deep lung.
  - Passing through bronchial secretions: These crackles occur in the proximal lung.
- Wheezing: These are continuous aperiodic vibrations that appear in the bronchial terminations. They are classified according to frequency and occurrence in the respiratory cycle.
- Rhonchi: These are low frequency polyphonic wheezes that indicate secretions in proximal airways.

- Noises at a distance:
  - Stridor: Stridor is an abnormal respiratory sound characterized by high-pitched and high frequency. It is produced by the vibration of the upper airway structures, especially during inspiration. Its presence indicates a partial or complete obstruction of the airway, from the nose to the middle of the trachea. Inspiratory and expiratory stridor is an important clinical sign suggesting severe airway obstruction. It can be caused by a variety of factors, including (19).
    - Infections: Such as laryngitis, which may be viral (e.g., due to parainfluenza virus), bacterial or other microorganism.
    - Allergies: Allergic reactions that cause inflammation of the upper respiratory tract.
    - Trauma: Injuries to the upper airway causing swelling or narrowing of the respiratory structures.
    - Congenital conditions: Anatomical abnormalities present from birth that affect the size or shape of the airways.

      It is important to note that stridor can be a sign of medical emergency, especially if accompanied by severe respiratory distress. In such cases, medical attention should be sought immediately to evaluate and treat the airway obstruction and ensure adequate oxygenation and ventilation.

The auscultation sequence for the posterior and anterior face of the thorax will be as follows (4):

- Rear face:
    - 1-2 Inferior lobe: inferior segment
    - 3-4 Inferior lobe: lateral segment
    - 5-6 Inferior lobe: apical segment
    - 7 Superior lobe: apical segment
    - 8 Superior lobe: apical/posterior segment
- Anterior face:
    - 9-10 Inferior lobe: anterior segment
    - 11 Median lobe
    - 12 Superior lobe: Ligula
    - 13-14 Superior lobe: anterior segment
    - 15-16 Superior lobe: apical segment

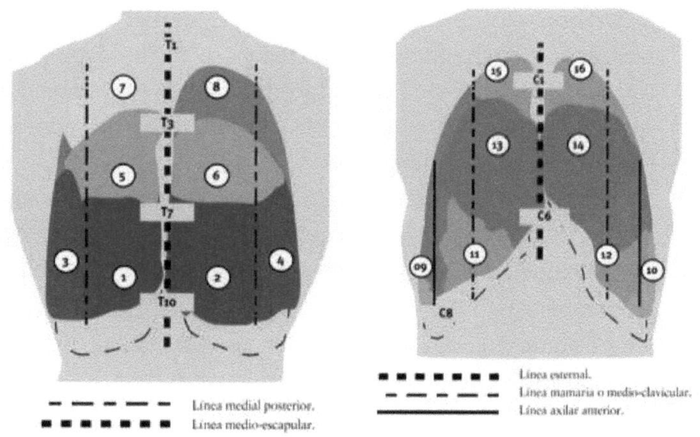

Auscultation sequence posterior thorax (left) and anterior thorax (right) (4).

3.1.6. Body plethysmography.

Body plethysmography is a procedure used to measure functional residual capacity (FRC) and airway resistance (Raw). It consists of a system that includes an airtight cabinet where the subject sits, two manometers to measure pressures, a flow meter connected to a pneumotachographic head through which the individual breathes, and an electric valve that closes during the measurement. The subject is placed inside the airtight cabinet and breathes through the pneumotachograph, which records the mouth pressure equated to the alveolar pressure. After a few minutes of normal breathing, the mouthpiece is closed when the patient exhales completely. The patient then attempts to inhale with the mouthpiece closed, which temporarily increases the pressure inside the box. The pressure inside the cabinet is recorded by another manometer. At the end of expiration, the alveolar pressure and the pressure inside the box are equal, and the intrathoracic gas volume is similar to the CRF. The volume inside the plethysmograph is known (23).

This procedure is used to measure total lung capacity and airway resistance, as well as to determine residual volume. It also helps in the diagnosis of obstructive airway disorders (23).

The indications for measurement cover various clinical situations (24):

- Early detection of airflow limitation, especially in cases at risk of developing chronic obstructive pulmonary disease, such as middle-aged women with alpha1-antitrypsin deficiency.
- Determine "trapped gas" in cases of specific lung diseases.
- To establish the diagnosis of restrictive ventilatory impairment and characterize the pattern of functional impairment in these diseases.
- In cases of suspected combined obstructive and restrictive impairment, volume measurement can confirm the restriction and distinguish between them, as well as provide a quantitative measure of their severity.
- To detect the response of lung volumes to bronchodilator testing and monitor the response to therapeutic interventions.
- Establish a prognosis, assess surgical risk and evaluate incapacity for work.
- Assist in the interpretation of other volume-dependent scans.
- Quantify the unventilated airspace by the difference between the functional residual capacity measured by plethysmography and the capacity assessed by helium dilution.

Contraindications are mainly relative and are related to the performance of the forced spirometry that usually accompanies this examination. Some of them include (24):

- Lack of patient understanding or cooperation
- Recent hemoptysis
- Pneumothorax treated with thoracic drainage
- Thoracic, abdominal or cerebral aneurysm
- Unstable cardiovascular pathology
- Recent ocular surgery,
- Acute illness that may interfere with the test,
- Recent chest or abdominal surgery
- Tracheostomized patients without airtight connection to the system
- Destructive lesions of the facial mass that allow gas leakage,
- Factors limiting the patient's access to the plethysmographic booth, such as claustrophobia or the need for supplemental oxygen and intravenous fluids that cannot be temporarily interrupted.

3.2.   Assessment of the respiratory patient.
3.2.1. Medical history.

The process of taking a medical history is fundamental in any Respiratory Physiotherapy intervention, a well elaborated medical history has the potential to provide an accurate diagnosis in approximately 75% of the cases. In addition, the data collected during the anamnesis guides the physical examination and may reduce the need for additional complementary tests. It also provides crucial information for selecting appropriate treatment techniques, evaluating the patient's evolution and determining the efficacy of the interventions performed. In addition, it allows an objective and scientific discussion of the results obtained. There are several clinical history models, among them (19):

- Chronological Medical History: follows the patient's evolution in chronological order, traditionally used in hospital settings.
- Health Problem Oriented Medical Record (HCOPP): Focuses on the patient's health problems and their relevance to the physician or patient.

- Protocolized Clinical History: uses closed questions and is used in specific diseases, such as anesthesiology.

When preparing a clinical history, we will set some objectives, these are (19):

- Organize the information in a way that facilitates the understanding of the problem and the identification of the objectives.
- Ensure continuity by transferring all relevant information to the medical record.
- Ensure quality of care by objectifying information, which can also serve as a legal document if necessary.

The information should be action-oriented, so it is crucial to select the relevant data and provide the necessary information. At the very least, the clinical history should include (19):

- Administrative data of the patient and the responsible physiotherapist.
- Personal and family history, etiological diagnosis, current pharmacology, allergies, smoking habits, and current symptoms.
- Use of home respiratory therapy, such as noninvasive mechanical ventilation or supplemental oxygen.
- Initial examination and physiotherapeutic diagnosis.
- Therapeutic objectives and treatment plan, including the number of sessions planned and contraindications.
- Record of the evolution and any relevant incident.
- Final assessment to prepare the discharge report.

3.2.2. Physical and Functional Exploration.
– Static observation of the thorax:

The thorax is anatomically divided into four faces: anterior, posterior and two lateral, and is evaluated by means of anatomical reference lines such as the anterior axillary line, the midclavicular line, the mid-sternal line, the third rib and the eighth rib, which help to detect possible deviations. Two types of thorax are distinguished: long and narrow, with the vertical axis longer than the transverse axis, and short and wide, with the vertical axis shorter than the transverse axis. Morphological alterations of the thorax can affect its form and function (23):

- Barrel chest: Increased anteroposterior diameter and horizontalized ribs, characteristic of pulmonary emphysema.
- Pectum excavatum: Sinking of the anterior part of the thorax, especially the sternum, can limit costal mobility and compress the left lung.
- Pectum carinatum: forward protrusion of the sternum, commonly associated with asthma.
- Paralytic thorax: Flattened, with oblique ribs downward, associated with weakness of the respiratory musculature.
- Asymmetric thorax: Loss of lateral symmetry of the thorax, associated with scoliosis and atelectasis.
- Kyphotic thorax: Limitation of rib mobility due to excessive backward curvature.
- Scoliotic thorax: Asymmetry in rib mobility due to scoliosis.
- Rachitic thorax: inelastic ribs and palpable spherical prominences at the chondro-costal junction, with bulky abdomen.
- Skirt chest: Circular narrowing in the pectorals with widening in the lower part, associated with asthma in young people.
- Pleuritic chest: Characteristic of pleural effusion, with bulging of the costal cartilages on the affected side and flattening on the healthy side.

- Dynamic assessment of the thorax:

An assessment of how the rib cage moves in the sagittal and frontal planes is performed by asking the patient to breathe in a habitual manner. From a frontal approach, the pattern of movement in the lower thorax is primarily examined, since it is more visible, while, from a sagittal perspective, it is determined whether breathing is predominantly performed with movement of the upper thorax or by involvement of the abdomen and diaphragm. Therefore, in relation to the respiratory pattern, the following aspects are considered (25):

- Type of breathing pattern: either upper costal, lower costal or abdomino-diaphragmatic.
- Intensity of ventilation: whether deep or shallow.
- Thoracic-abdominal coordination: it is observed how both the thorax and the abdomen expand during inspiration. Possible diaphragmatic dysfunctions that may alter this process are identified.
- Ventilatory synergies: Abnormal movements associated with breathing are assessed, such as the pulling of the accessory respiratory muscles or the active contraction of the abdominal muscles. We also find Hoover's sign, where it is evaluated if during inspiration there is a paradoxical movement in the ribs, that is, if the transverse diameter decreases instead of increasing. This may indicate diaphragmatic dysfunction or other irregularities in respiratory mechanics.
- Inspiration-expiration time ratio: Normally, the ratio between inspiration and expiration time is 1:2, which means that the time dedicated to expiration is twice the time dedicated to inspiration.
- Ventilatory mode: This refers to the way in which ventilation is performed, either by the nose, by the nose and mouth, or only by the mouth.
- Respiratory rate: The number of breaths per minute. Under normal conditions, an adult breathes between 12 and 15 times per minute at rest. Alterations in respiratory rate may include:
  - Tachypnea: Increased respiratory rate, with rapid and shallow respirations (more than 24 breaths per minute).
  - Bradypnea: Decrease in respiratory rate (less than 10 breaths per minute).
  - Apnea: Periods without breathing.
  - Polypnea: Increase in both respiratory depth and respiratory rate.

- Hyperpnea or bathypnea: Increased depth of respiratory movements.
- Hypopnea: Shallow breathing with decreased amplitude.
- Alterations of respiratory rhythms:
  - Kussmaul Breathing: Characterized by a wide, deep, noisy inspiration followed by a brief pause, then a short, gasping exhalation. Usually seen in patients with diabetic acidosis and coma.

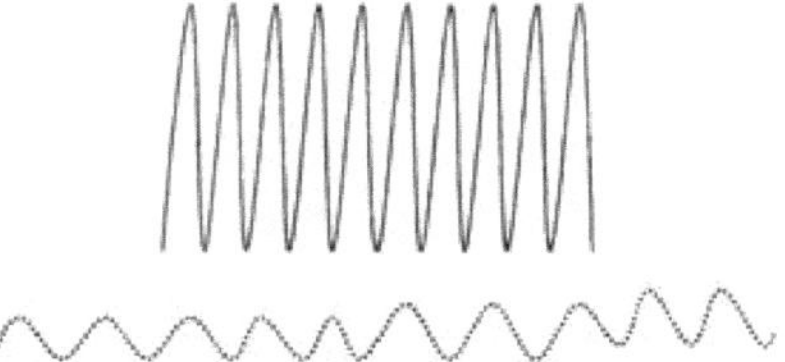

Figure 12. Schematic representation of Kussmaul's respiration (The dotted line represents the normal pattern) (23).

  - Cheyne Stokes respiration: It is characterized by a series of breaths of increasing and decreasing depth followed by a period of apnea. It may be seen in patients with various medical conditions, such as heart failure, coma, etc.

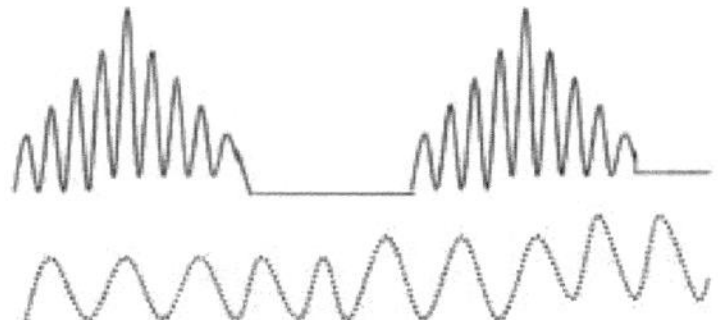

Figure 13. Schematic representation of Cheyne Stokes respiration (the dotted line represents the normal pattern) (23).

  - Biot respiration: Irregular respirations of variable depth interrupted by intervals of apnea. It is observed in preagonic states and in cases of lesions in the respiratory center.

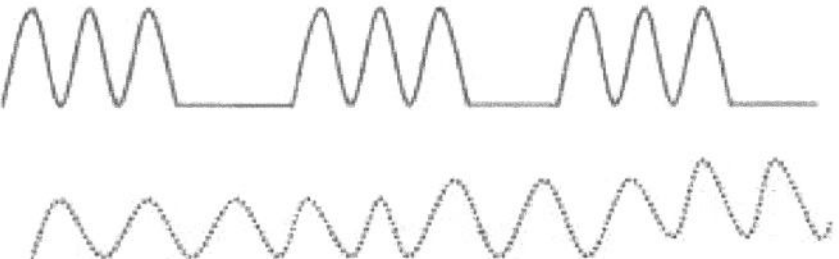

Figure 14. Schematic representation of Biot's respiration (The dotted line represents the normal pattern) (23).

- Sighing, Nervous or Dysphrenic Breathing: It consists of a deep and noisy inspiration followed by a prolonged exhalation, accompanied by sensations of anguish and precordial oppression. It may be associated with emotional problems, anxiety, among others.
- Ondine respiration: It is characterized by transient losses of automatic respiration, and may be observed in acute lesions of the medulla oblongata or upper cervical cord.
- Sleep apnea: Refers to pauses in breathing during sleep, with intense inspiratory sounds at the end of the apnea. This disorder can result in unrefreshing sleep.
- Hiccups: These are abrupt contractions of the diaphragm that produce a characteristic sound when air passes through the glottis.

To assess the mobility of the thorax, a manual exploration of the thorax is performed using the techniques of upper and lower amplexation, as well as amplexion. The maneuvers are detailed below:

- In upper amplexation, the hands are positioned over the supraclavicular hollows, with the thumbs on the spinous processes and the middle and index fingers on the clavicles. It is important to apply gentle pressure without exerting force to allow the thorax to move freely.
- For lower amplexation, the hands are placed symmetrically at the level of the infrascapular line, with the thumbs away from the spine.
- In amplexion: It allows to determine the amplitude of the respiratory movement in the anteroposterior direction of each hemithorax. One hand is placed on the anterior and the other on

the posterior side of each side of the thorax, both upper and lower. During inspiration and deep expiration, both hemithoraxes are observed to expand simultaneously and with equal amplitude in both respiratory phases.

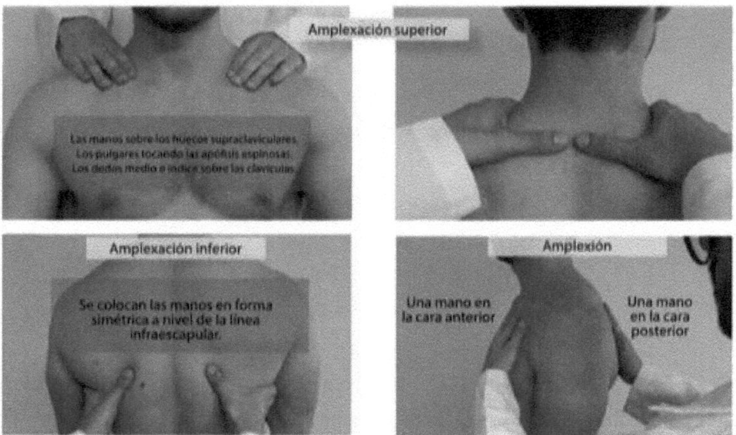

Figure 15. Manual exploration of the thorax in amplexation maneuvers (25).

- Thoracic mobility assessment can also be performed considering Keith's zones. The physical therapist will position the hands with thumbs facing each other on the area to be assessed. The patient will then be asked to perform deep inhalations and exhalations. The mobility of the rib cage will be evaluated according to the separation between both thumbs, observing if it occurs synchronously or if blockages or other anomalies are present. During the assessment, the patient is instructed to breathe in slowly and deeply, while observing the separation between the two thumbs of the physical therapist. A minimum separation of 1 cm is considered normal and can be as small as 3-5 cm. In addition, attention is paid to any asymmetry in the movement with respect to the reference line, where a minimum difference of 0.5 cm may be significant for the evaluation. The areas are distributed as follows (9):
    - Zone 1: Includes the first rib and the sternal manubrium.

- Zone 2: Comprises the upper ribs, from the second to the sixth rib.
- Zone 3: Encompasses the lower ribs, from the seventh to the tenth.
- Zone 4: Encompasses the floating ribs that are not functionally related to the thorax.

An instrumental assessment of the thorax is performed, where the expansion capacity of the thoracic cage is evaluated, using a cirtometer or a Rosenthal tape. Symmetrical points, one anterior and one posterior, are marked on the thorax, specifically at the level of the base of the thorax (xiphoid thoracometry) and in the upper third of the thorax (upper axillary thoracometry). Then, a semicircle is drawn on a sheet of paper joining the two marked points. The patient is instructed to perform a deep costal inspiration, followed by a deep exhalation. This provides a graphic representation of the cross-sectional view, allowing changes in both rib statics and dynamics to be observed. This assessment not only provides a visualization of thoracic expansion, but also facilitates tailored functional re-education, which can help adjust mobility in the area of interest as needed (9).

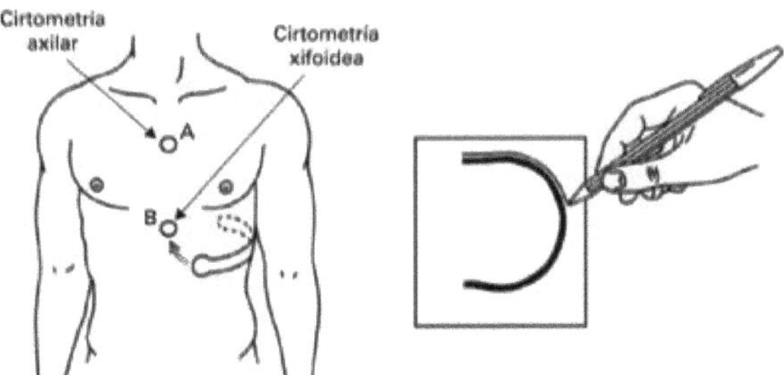

Figure 16. Thorax evaluation with cirtometer (26).

Conditions for cirtometry (26):

- The patient's breathing should be of the costal type, avoiding abdominal breathing.
- Inspiration and expiration should have the same intensity; it is recommended that the patient practices several times before the measurement.

- The landmarks marked on the thorax should be symmetrical.
- The cirtometer should join the anterior and posterior points perpendicular to the spine. In addition, the points on the same side of the thorax should be aligned vertically and in the midline.
- For optimal results, the measurement should be performed with the patient standing and the torso naked, although this may vary depending on the patient's condition.
- If the measurement is correct, the two semicircles corresponding to each hemithorax should continue each other, coinciding at their points.

If we perform a dynamic diaphragmatic assessment, we will use radiography or dynamic radioscopy to evaluate the expansion capacity of the abdominal area by means of three main measures (26):

- The brake-inspiratory index records the maximum displacement of the diaphragm in the caudal direction. It is calculated by measuring the distance between the centerline of the two diaphragmatic paths during normal breathing and the travel of the diaphragm during a maximal inspiration.
- The brake-expiratory index quantifies the maximum displacement of the diaphragm in the cranial direction. It is obtained by measuring the distance between the centerline of the two diaphragmatic paths during normal breathing and the path of the diaphragm during maximal expiration.
- The brake-kinetic index, or total path, represents the maximum total displacement of the diaphragm. It is calculated by measuring the distance between the maximum cranial position and the maximum caudal position of the diaphragm.

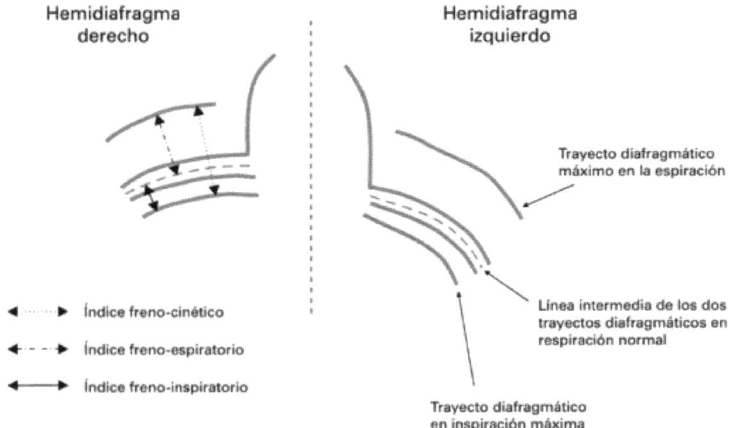

Figure 17. Representation of the 3 indices of diaphragmatic dynamic assessment (26).

These indices may vary according to the patient's position. In the standing position, the brake-expiratory index predominates, while in the supine position the brake-inspiratory index predominates. It is therefore advisable to perform all measurements in the same position for an accurate comparison of the results obtained in each treatment. In a healthy individual, diaphragmatic mobility can reach up to 10 cm (26).

- Assessment of the respiratory musculature:

The joints of the ribs, vertebrae and sternum limit the specific mobility of the thorax during respiration. With the action of the muscles, the ribs move to modify the vertical, transverse and anteroposterior diameters of the thorax. During inspiration, most of the respiratory muscles are active, generating three phases of increased thoracic dimension through contraction of the diaphragm (27):

- In the first phase, the diaphragmatic domes flatten, increasing the vertical diameter of the thorax.

- In the second phase, the lower ribs are elevated and horizontalized, increasing the transverse diameter, known as the "bucket-handle" movement.
- In the third phase, elevation of the upper ribs and sternum occurs, increasing the anteroposterior diameter, called "pump lever" movement.

During inspiration, the diaphragm contracts, increasing lung volume and creating a more negative intrapleural pressure, which prevents lung collapse. Normal expiration is passive due to the elasticity of the chest wall and lung parenchyma, and the relaxation of the inspiratory muscles. However, in activities that require a high energy demand, such as laughing, singing or physical activity, the expiratory muscles are activated. The bronchi shorten, the internal intercostal muscles pull the ribs downward and inward, while the abdominal muscles increase intra-abdominal pressure, displacing the diaphragm upward (27).

The main respiratory muscles can be classified into two groups according to their predominant function: inspiratory or expiratory (26).

- Fundamentally inspiratory muscles:
  - Sternocleidomastoid
  - Pectoralis major and minor
  - Superior posterior serratus
  - Trapeze
  - Anterior and middle scalenes
  - External intercostals
- Fundamentally expiratory muscles:
  - Internal intercostals
  - Rectus abdominis
  - Oblique abdominal muscles
  - Serrate minor
  - Transversus abdominis

Each of these muscles plays a specific role during respiration, contributing to the movement of the ribs, the expansion and contraction of the thorax, and the change in lung volume necessary for gas exchange.

We can distinguish other types of musculature that influence respiration such as (26):

- The external intercostal muscles, along with the parasternal portion of the internal intercostals, are considered primarily inspiratory. During inspiration, the external intercostals contract and activate in the upper intercostal spaces in a craniocaudal sequence. On the other hand, the internal intercostals, classically considered expiratory muscles, contract during expiration in the lower intercostal spaces with a caudocranial sequential activation. Both groups are innervated by the intercostal nerves. Although their exact contribution to respiratory mechanics is not completely clear and may be primarily postural, they also play important roles in trunk rotation.
- Accessory muscles are inactive during resting respiration in normal individuals, but can be activated under certain conditions. They are divided into:
    - Accessory muscles of inspiration: This group includes muscles that elevate the ribs, such as the pectoralis major, pectoralis minor, trapezius, serratus, and sternocleidomastoid, as well as some laryngeal muscles. These muscles have a relevant role in the ventilation of people with chronic obstructive pulmonary disease (COPD). Among them, the sternocleidomastoid is the one that contributes most to respiratory mechanics, as evidenced in tetraplegic patients with high spinal cord injuries, where hypertrophy and forceful contraction during inspiration are observed.
    - Accessory expiratory muscle: Represented by the sternocostal or triangular sternum muscle, it acts when the functional residual capacity decreases and in spontaneous forced expiratory maneuvers, such as coughing and laughing.

The main muscle actions that happen during dynamic breathing can be divided into:

- Dynamic type inspiration: The scalenes, from their upper fixed point on the cervical spine, posteriorize the first two ribs, thus ensuring the correct position of the angle of Louis and preventing paradoxical inspiratory depression of the upper thorax. In addition, they activate the external intercostal muscles, whose fibers are similarly oriented and extend throughout the intercostal space, protecting the rib cage from collapse due to atmospheric pressure. Dorsally, the supracostals, which extend from the cervical vertebrae to the lower ribs, have a similar fiber direction to the external intercostals and scalenes. They extend into the transvers spinous and hold the lesser rib arm in place, allowing its elevation and preventing its downward subluxation. This contributes to maintain the good orientation of the greater rib arm. At the lumbar level, the transversus spinosus transmits tension to the vertebral insertions of the transversus abdominis, preparing it to respond to the contraction of the diaphragm. It is suggested that the transverse spinous gives a fixed point to the phrenic center, although some argue that it is primarily the endothoracic fascia that serves this function. The transversus abdominis controls intra-abdominal pressure, directing it upward during inspiration, which contributes to trunk straightening and prevents excessive pressure on the lesser pelvis. The sternal triangle, an extension of the transverse abdominis, joins the sternum and costal cartilages, suspending the sternum in the rib cage and limiting excessive rib elevation. The tonicity of the rectus abdominis helps keep the sternum vertical, while the transverse abdominis controls the opening of Charpy's angle and excessive elevation of the lower thorax, preventing stemo-costal dissociation during inspiration. Once everything is in place, the diaphragm elevates the symphysis rib cage, thus increasing all thoracic diameters from a simple rib cage elevation movement (27).

- Dynamic exhalation: In this phase, known as thoracic compliance, the muscles relax, returning the thoracic cage to its initial position. This relaxation is directly related to the elasticity of the anatomical elements of the thorax and lungs. To better understand this phenomenon, it is important to understand costal physiology. The costal arch articulates posteriorly with the intervertebral disc and the transverse process of the lower vertebra, and anteriorly with the sternum through the costal cartilage. The ribs rotate on themselves at the level of their disc insertion, while resting on the transverse process that supports them on the outside. Observing the 4th to 10th costal arches, it can be noted that they are twisted on themselves, which means that their two extremities are in opposite rotation. This twisting can be illustrated with the analogy of an arm: by externally rotating the arm from the root and then bending it, the shape of a costal arch is simulated, showing how internal and external rotation are combined in the movement. During inspiration, the internal rotation of the distal limb of the costal arch is accentuated, as is the external rotation of its proximal limb, causing the rib to twist further on itself. This keeps the sternum vertical and opposes the excessive tonicity of the posterior muscles, maintaining the dorsal octave as the vertex of the kyphosis. The sternum is held in good position by the tonicity of the rectus abdominis, while the triangular sternum supports the costal cartilages. During inspiration, the ribs tense this muscle with their lifting movement and distal internal rotation, which, together with the elasticity of the costal cartilages, brings the anterior thorax downward. Except in forced expiration, the expiratory time is passive, which means that the muscles are not active during this phase (27).

- Methods of assessment of the respiratory musculature:

Strength and endurance are two fundamental properties of any muscle, including respiratory muscles. Strength refers to the maximum contractile capacity of a muscle, and depends on factors such as muscle mass, transverse size of the muscle, intramuscular and intermuscular coordination, and muscle composition. On the other hand, endurance is defined as the ability to sustain an effort for a prolonged period of time below the maximum, and is related to the aerobic capacity of the muscle. When a muscle cannot adequately fulfill its function, we speak of muscle dysfunction. Fatigue occurs when there is a deficit of muscular endurance, while muscular weakness refers to a deficit of muscular strength (20).

The evaluation of the respiratory musculature can be performed analytically, focusing on a specific muscle, or globally, evaluating all the respiratory musculature together. The analytical evaluation can be manual or instrumental. On the other hand, global assessment can be carried out using methods to measure muscle strength, such as peak inspiratory pressure (MIP), peak expiratory pressure (PEM), nasal inspiratory fast inspiratory pressure (SNIP), and methods to measure muscle endurance, such as maximal voluntary ventilation (MVV) (20).

The methods of evaluation of the respiratory musculature can be both analytical and global. Among the analytical methods, manual and instrumental methods can be distinguished (20):

- Manual analytical methods: These are mainly used to evaluate the diaphragm, the main respiratory muscle. In this method, one hand is placed on the epigastric angle to detect if there is a descent of the diaphragmatic domes during inspiration, while the other hand is placed on the abdomen to check for abdominal expansion due to caudal displacement of the diaphragm and abdominal viscera.
- Instrumental analytical methods: Respiratory muscle strength is assessed in terms of pressure. Differential transducers are used to measure respiratory pressures, such as transdiaphragmatic pressure (TDP), which is the difference between esophageal pressure (EP) and gastric pressure (GP). This measurement can be performed voluntarily or involuntarily, by stimulation of the phrenic nerve. In addition, electromyographic studies with electrodes on the respiratory muscles can be used to evaluate their activity.
- Muscle strength specific test: It is performed by measuring Maximal Respiratory Pressures (MPR), which include inspiratory (MIP) and maximal expiratory pressures (MEP). The patient generates the maximal inspiratory pressure from the residual volume and the maximal expiratory pressure from the total lung capacity, using equipment that measures pressure
- Non-specific test of respiratory muscular endurance: maximal voluntary ventilation (MVV). It consists of performing maximum ventilation for 15 seconds, with the fastest and deepest breathing possible, while tidal volume, respiratory frequency and respiratory

pattern are recorded. It is non-specific because it evaluates both inspiratory and expiratory musculature.

- Specific respiratory muscle endurance tests: These involve mechanical overload of the respiratory muscles, using systems such as the resisted or threshold opening valve system, applying incremental or constant respiratory loads. These tests focus on specifically assessing respiratory muscle endurance.

- Percussion:

The most commonly used percussion technique in the physical examination of the thorax is the digitodigital or Gerhart technique. It consists of indirectly tapping with one or two fingers on the second phalanx of the middle finger of the hand. When this percussion is performed on the thoracic areas corresponding to the lung, a normally clear sound is produced, which is known as pulmonary clear. The sounds that can be heard during percussion can vary and provide information about the condition of the lungs and underlying structures (9):

- Decreased resonance: Characterized by a dull sound during percussion. This may indicate non-aerated areas in the lung, as occurs in conditions such as pneumonectomy (surgical removal of an entire lung), pleural effusion, atelectasis (partial or complete collapse of a lung) or pulmonary consolidation.
- Increased resonance: This is characterized by a more hollow or tympanic sound during percussion. This may indicate areas of increased air in the lung, as occurs in pneumothorax (accumulation of air in the pleural space) or pulmonary emphysema (abnormal enlargement of the air spaces distal to the terminal bronchioles, with destruction of the lung parenchyma).

Chest percussion is an important tool in the physical examination to assess lung health and can provide important clues to various respiratory conditions. However, it is important to remember that the interpretation of percussive sounds must be integrated with other clinical findings and diagnostic tests to obtain an accurate diagnosis (9).

3.2.3. Assessment of the signs and symptoms of the patient with respiratory pathology.

- Assessment of dyspnea:

Dyspnea is described as a subjective experience of respiratory distress consisting of distinct qualitative sensations that vary both in intensity and in their unpleasantness, emotionality, and behavioral significance. This definition highlights that dyspnea goes beyond simply being a respiratory sensation; it can involve emotional and psychological aspects, as well as have a significant impact on the individual's behavior. It is important to keep in mind that dyspnea can be a major symptom in a variety of diseases, not only of the respiratory system, but also of the cardiovascular or neuromuscular system. In fact, on many occasions, dyspnea is the symptom that leads patients with pulmonary disease to seek medical attention. Since dyspnea can manifest in a variety of ways and have multiple underlying causes, it is crucial to perform a thorough evaluation to identify the specific cause and provide the appropriate treatment to alleviate the symptom and improve the patient's quality of life (28).

The anamnesis is fundamental to identify the form of dyspnea presentation and can guide the study and diagnosis of dyspnea. Some common forms of dyspnea include (28):

- Dyspnea on exertion: It appears during physical activities and can be classified according to the intensity of the effort made.
- Dyspnea at rest: It manifests itself even in the absence of any physical exertion.
- Orthopnea: Dyspnea that occurs in the dorsal decubitus position and forces the patient to sit or sit up to relieve it. It may be related to heart failure or other respiratory pathologies.
- Paroxysmal nocturnal dyspnea: The patient wakes up with a choking sensation, which forces him/her to get up, leave the bed or open windows. It is usually observed in cases of heart failure.
- Platypnea: It is characterized by dyspnea in the standing position that is relieved by adopting the supine position. It may be

associated with hepato-pulmonary syndrome, pulmonary arteriovenous fistulas or cardiac circuit problems.

- Trepopnea: A form of dyspnea in which there is intolerance to lateral decubitus, usually due to contralateral pleural effusion or cardiac malformation.
- Hyperventilation: Corresponds to rapid and deep breathing, which may be a response to anxiety or panic attacks.
- Tachypnea: Increased respiratory rate, usually above 25 breaths per minute.
- Polypnea: Fast and shallow breathing.
- Periodic or Cheyne-Stokes breathing: It is characterized by alternating periods of apnea with periods of breathing that gradually increase in frequency and then decrease until a new apnea. It may be of cardiac or cerebral origin or related to the administration of certain drugs.

Each type of dyspnea may indicate different underlying conditions, so it is important to perform a thorough evaluation to determine the exact cause and plan appropriate treatment.

In addition to assessing the intensity of dyspnea, it is important to consider other aspects, such as (28):

- Intensity: Both at rest and during exertion.
- Onset: It can be paroxysmal (sudden and episodic onset), inspiratory (due to upper airway stenosis) or expiratory (due to small bronchial stenosis).
- Association with the position adopted: For example, orthopnea (improved sitting and standing) or platypnea (associated with standing).
- Presence of specific triggering factors: Such as temperature changes, exercise, body position, etc.
- Accompanying respiratory sounds.
- Variations throughout the day: There may be fluctuations in the intensity of dyspnea at different times of the day.

Dyspnea can be quantified by means of measurement scales. These scales allow the magnitude of the symptom and its changes to be evaluated. The dyspnea value can be used as a reliable tool to determine exercise intensity. It is important to select the most appropriate rating scale for each patient and situation, preferably one that is translated and validated in the language and sociocultural context of the population under study. There are two main types of dyspnea scales (28):

- One-dimensional scales (28):
  - The Modified Medical Research Council Scale (mMRC) is a widely used tool for assessing dyspnea in patients with respiratory disease, especially chronic obstructive pulmonary disease (COPD). This scale, proposed by the British society in the 1960s, was originally graded from 1 to 5, with a lower score indicating less limitation due to dyspnea. However, nowadays, the mMRC scale is more frequently used with a grading of 0 to 4, which allows greater sensitivity in the assessment of dyspnea. This scale is easy to administer and has been recommended by the Spanish Society of Pneumology and Thoracic Surgery (SEPAR) for the evaluation of obstructive diseases such as COPD. The GOLD (Global Initiative for Chronic Obstructive Lung Disease) classification uses the mMRC as one of the parameters to categorize the severity of COPD, along with others such as lung function measured by spirometry (FEV1). However, it is important to keep in mind that mMRC is a unidimensional scale, which means that it may be limited in capturing subtle changes in dyspnea after therapeutic interventions.

Medical Research Council Questionnaire		
1. If you are unable to walk for reasons other than your heart or lungs, check the box.	YES	NO
2. Are you short of breath walking fast on the flat or going up a gentle slope?		

3. Do you become fatigued or short of breath when walking on the plain at other people's normal pace?
4. Do you have to stop to catch your breath when walking at your own pace on the plain?
5. Are you short of breath just getting dressed or getting up?

Table 7. Medical Research Council questionnaire to assess the magnitude of dyspnea (28).

- The modified Borg Scale is a tool for assessing perceived exertion, especially dyspnea, during exercise. This scale uses a graduation from 0 to 10, where 0 represents the absence of dyspnea and 10 indicates the maximum sensation of dyspnea. Although originally based on a twenty-level scale, the modified version simplifies this range to ten levels. Although not a quantitative scale in the strict sense, values have been shown to increase linearly with physiological measurements such as heart rate and oxygen consumption as exercise intensity increases.

Modified Borg Scale	
10	Maximum
9	Very, very severe
8	
7	Very severe
6	
5	Severa
4	Somewhat severe
3	Moderate
2	Slight
1	Very Slight
0,5	Very, very mild
0	Null

Table 8. Modified Borg scale to assess perceived exertion.

- The Sadoul Scale is another internationally validated tool that assesses dyspnea on a grading from 0 to 5 degrees, where a minimum score indicates no dyspnea. This scale also assesses the level of exertion required to trigger dyspnea and health-related quality of life.

- The Visual Analog Scale (VAS) consists of a 100 mm straight line where one end represents the absence of dyspnea and the other end represents the maximum dyspnea. The patient marks on the line the point that reflects his or her perception of dyspnea.
- The ATS (American Thoracic Society) Dyspnea Scale uses a grading from 0 to 4, with the lowest score indicating no dyspnea except during strenuous exercise. Each of these scales provides a way to measure and communicate the intensity of dyspnea in an objective and standardized manner.

- Multidimensional: They include the sensation of dyspnea during various activities of daily living. Usually used more in research, we find different scales such as (28):
  - The Mahler Baseline Dyspnea Index (BMDI) is a scale that assesses three dimensions of dyspnea at a specific time point: task difficulty, exertional intensity, and functional impairment. Each dimension is scored on a scale from 0 (absent) to 4 (very intense), and the total score ranges from 0 to 12, where a higher score indicates a greater perception of dyspnea.

MAHLER BASAL INDEX (MBI)	
1. MAGNITUDE OF THE TASK.	
Grade 4	Dyspnea only with extraordinary activity such as heavy load or light load on slope. No dyspnea with ordinary tasks.
Grade 3	Dyspnea with major activities, such as steep slopes, more than three flights of stairs or moderate overhead loading.
Grade 2	Dyspnea with activities such as light slopes, less than three flights of stairs or light overhead loading.
Grade 1	Dyspnea on small efforts, walking, washing or standing.
Grade 0	Dyspnea at rest, sitting or lying down.
2. FUNCTIONAL INCAPACITY	
Grade 4	Not incapacitated; performs activities and occupations without dyspnea.
Grade 3	Slight incapacity; reduction, although not abandonment, of some habitual activity.
Grade 2	Moderate disability; abandonment of some usual activity due to dyspnea.

Grade 1	Severe disability; she has abandoned most of her usual activities because of dyspnea.
Grade 0	Very severe disability; has abandoned all usual activities due to dyspnea.
3. MAGNITUDE OF THE EFFORT	
Grade 4	Only heavy exertion causes dyspnea. No ordinary exertional dyspnea.
Grade 3	Dyspnea with somewhat greater than ordinary exertion. The tasks can be done without rest.
Grade 2	Dyspnea with moderate efforts. Tasks done with occasional breaks.
Grade 1	Dyspnea of small efforts. Tasks performed with frequent breaks.
Grade 0	Dyspnea at rest, sitting or lying down.

Table 9. Mahler's baseline index (28).

- The San Diego Short-Course Respiratory Questionnaire (UCSDQ) assesses dyspnea during 21 different activities on a 6-point scale, allowing for a detailed assessment of dyspnea in a variety of everyday situations.
- The Dyspnea Dimension of the Chronic Respiratory Disease Questionnaire is part of a larger questionnaire that assesses dyspnea in five essential activities of daily living (ADLs) during the past two weeks. Dyspnea is scored on a 7-point scale for each activity, providing a detailed measure of perceived dyspnea in different settings and activities.

- Assessment of cough:

Cough is a common symptom in respiratory patients and can be reflex or voluntary, composed of three phases: inspiratory, compressive and expiratory. An effective cough is one that succeeds in removing secretions, and its efficacy can be assessed by strength testing. It is triggered by a deep inhalation followed by glottal closure and abrupt expulsion at high velocity, using 60% to 80% of total lung capacity. The stimuli that activate this reflex can be chemical or mechanical, with receptors located in different areas of the respiratory tract. The bronchial mucosa, especially in the posterior part of the larynx and epiglottis, followed by the trachea and main bronchi, is particularly sensitive to these stimuli, mainly to prevent bronchial aspiration. It is important to differentiate between the types of cough, as this may influence the indication for treatment with Respiratory Physiotherapy. There are two main types of cough: productive and unproductive. Productive cough, which produces mouth crackles, indicates the presence of proximal secretions and is an indication for respiratory physiotherapy with the aim of removing secretions. In contrast, unproductive cough, which may be dry, irritative or spasmodic, does not benefit from respiratory physiotherapy (28).

The effectiveness of coughing is assessed by measuring the thrust velocity or peak cough flow (PCF). A device called a flow meter, such as the Miniwright or peak flow meter, is used to measure PCF when coughing through the device. PCF values between 360 and 1200 L/min are considered effective, whereas a PCF < 160 L/min indicates an ineffective cough and a PCF < 270 L/min increases the risk of respiratory morbidity. A cough is considered effective when the PCF is between 160 and 180 L/min. Ineffective cough may be caused primarily by weakness of the expiratory musculature, including the internal intercostals and abdominal musculature. This weakness can lead to impaired phonation and swallowing, increasing the risk of bronchoaspiration and eventually acute respiratory failure. Assisted cough is recommended for patients with a peak cough flow less than 270 L/min and/or with a Peak Expiratory Pressure (PEM) less than 60 cm H2O, a vital capacity less than 50% of its baseline value and a Peak Inspiratory Pressure (PIM) less than 80 cm H2O, applying instrumental assistance in inspiration. In addition to the intensity, frequency and timing of cough, it is important to consider its onset (acute or chronic) and the triggering circumstances, such as exertion or decubitus (28).

The Leicester Cough Questionnaire (LCQ) is a reliable and validated tool to assess chronic cough in children and adolescents with cystic fibrosis. This questionnaire assesses three domains: physical, psychological and social, allowing to measure the impact of cough on quality of life (28).

- Assessment of expectoration:

Expectoration is a physiological process by which material accumulated in the respiratory tract, mainly mucus, is expelled. Mucus normally has a quantity of about 10 ml per day. It is composed of two layers: a liquid layer (sol), which contains most of the cilia, and another thicker layer (gel), which transports particles and impurities and is displaced by the distal end of the cilia. When there is a malfunction in this cleaning system, mucus can accumulate, which favors the retention of secretions and increases the risk of respiratory infections. Sputum is the material expelled from the respiratory tract. When expectoration is abundant, the term "bronchorrhea" is used. This expectoration can vary in quantity and characteristics depending on the respiratory condition of the individual (28).

- Sputum evaluation:

Sputum assessment is an important part of the clinical evaluation of patients with respiratory conditions. Here are some aspects to consider when evaluating sputum (28):

- Origin: It should be determined whether the sputum comes from rhinopharyngeal or tracheobronchial secretions. This can be assessed by auscultation and by observing the behavior of the secretions during the application of various respiratory techniques.
- Frequency: It is important to quantify the amount of sputum produced by the patient during the day.
- Aspect: The macroscopic characteristics of the sputum are evaluated, such as color, volume, and viscosity. Some of the aspects to consider are:
- Color: May vary from serous (indicative of acute pulmonary edema) to purulent (indicative of infection).
- Volume: It can be measured using a graduated beaker to determine how much space the sputum occupies.

- Viscosity: The rheological property of viscosity is evaluated by observing how the sputum behaves when the vessel is inverted and laterally tilted.
- Filancia: Refers to the ability of sputum to form threads between two surfaces when trying to separate them.
- Microscopic analysis: In addition to macroscopic evaluation, microscopic, cytological and bacteriological analysis of sputum can be performed to identify possible pathogens or abnormal cells.

Sputum evaluation provides valuable information for the diagnosis and management of respiratory diseases, allowing the physician to make appropriate therapeutic decisions.

- Assessment of chest pain:

Assessment of chest pain is crucial to determine its underlying cause. Here is a description of the most common types of chest pain (28):

- Pain of joint and muscle structures: This type of pain is localized and is usually associated with problems in the joints or muscles of the chest. It may be worsened by local palpation or by moving certain parts of the body. Common examples include costochondritis, muscle strain and arthritis.
- Pleuritic pain: Refers to pain originating from the pleura, the membrane that lines the lungs and the interior of the thoracic cavity. This pain is of variable intensity and tends to worsen during deep inspiration, coughing or chest movements. It may be described as sharp, stabbing or cutting. Common causes include pleuritis, pneumonia, pulmonary embolism and pleural diseases such as pneumothorax.

Accurate identification of the type of chest pain can provide important clues as to the possible underlying cause and guide the appropriate treatment plan.

- Hemoptysis: Refers to the expulsion of blood through the mouth, which may occur as part of sputum. Hemoptysis is a serious symptom that may indicate conditions such as bronchopulmonary cancer, bronchiectasis or tuberculosis (28).

- Cyanosis: Cyanosis is the bluish coloration of the skin and mucous membranes due to hypoxemia, which may be due to low arterial oxygen saturation. Cyanosis is classified as central, which manifests in warm areas of the body, and peripheral, which is seen in cooler areas (28).
- Acropaquias: They are characterized by a painless enlargement of the distal ends of the fingers, also known as "clubbing" or digital hypoacrocytosis. They may be indicative of conditions such as bronchial neoplasms, bronchiectasis or pulmonary fibrosis (28).
- Asterixis or "flapping tremor": It is a clinical sign associated with hypoxemia and hypercapnia. It manifests as an alternating movement of flexion and extension of the wrists when the arms are extended, similar to flapping (28).
- Cor pulmonare: Refers to the structural and functional alteration of the right ventricle of the heart due to pulmonary hypertension unrelated to left or congenital heart disease. It can lead to right heart failure and is usually associated with chronic obstructive pulmonary diseases or acute pulmonary thromboembolism (28).

These aspects are important for the comprehensive evaluation of patients with respiratory diseases and may provide important clues for the diagnosis and proper management of these diseases.

- Radiological evaluation:

Interpreting a chest radiograph requires detailed knowledge of several technical and morphologic aspects. It is necessary to know (23):

- How the radiography was performed:
    - Projection: Understand the position and angle from which the radiograph was taken, either anteroposterior (AP) or posteroanterior (PA).
    - Degree of inspiration: Assess whether it is a full or partial inspiration, which may affect the position of the diaphragm and lung structures.
    - Sufficient contrast: Ensure adequate contrast between soft structures and bony tissues for better visualization.
- Reading of morphological alterations of the thorax:

- Identify signs of hyperinflation or restriction that may indicate conditions such as emphysema or pulmonary fibrosis.
- Recognition of pathological images:
  - Increased or decreased density or thickness of a structure, which may manifest as opacity or hyperclarity on the radiograph.
  - Recognize the association of these morphological changes with various pulmonary diseases.
- Assessment of airway obstruction: Identify signs of hyperinflation, such as horizontalized ribs, anteriorly displaced sternum, flattened diaphragm domes, among others. Observe specific radiographic features suggestive of airway obstruction, such as increased number of costal arches or "suspended heart" image.
- Assessment of altered external ventilatory mechanics: Look for signs of diaphragmatic insufficiency, such as an elevated diaphragmatic dome or a pinched costodiaphragmatic angle.

Keeping these aspects in mind is crucial for an accurate interpretation of a chest X-ray and can provide valuable information about the patient's lung health.

- Assessment of tolerance to physical exercise:

Stress testing is essential to assess cardiorespiratory fitness during exercise, especially in aerobic activities. This assessment is crucial to understand physical capacity and exercise tolerance, especially in people with chronic respiratory diseases such as COPD and mucoviscidosis. Oxygen consumption (VO2) is the main parameter used to define the functional capacity of an individual during an exercise test. A MET (metabolic equivalent) is defined as the oxygen consumption of a person at rest. One MET is equivalent to 3.5 ml of oxygen per kilogram of body weight per minute. This METs concept is used to provide a simplified and economical measure of maximal oxygen consumption (VO2max) (20).

- Incremental stress test: The cardiopulmonary exercise test (PCPE) is a comprehensive evaluation that allows examining the physiological response to exercise, involving the cardiovascular, respiratory, metabolic, musculoskeletal and neurosensory systems. From the clinical point of view, this test offers several utilities, such as the evaluation of exercise capacity, identification of limiting factors, functional follow-up of patients, evaluation of prognosis and response to treatments, among others. PCPE can be performed using a treadmill or an ergometer bicycle, and its main objective is to gradually increase energy requirements to assess the functional reserve of organs and systems during exercise. Indications for this test include dyspnea of unclear cause, quantification of disability, preoperative evaluation, treatment evaluation, exercise-induced asthma, and rehabilitation programs. It is considered the gold standard for assessing functional capacity. However, there are both absolute and relative contraindications to this test. Absolute contraindications include recent acute myocardial infarction, unstable angina, severe arrhythmias, among others, while relative contraindications include arterial hypertension, moderate heart disease, among others. The test is stopped if clinical signs such as falling oxygen saturation, cyanosis, severe dyspnea, central nervous system symptoms, electrocardiogram changes, among others, are present. This is done for patient safety reasons (20).

- Submaximal tests are useful tools for studying the physiological response of the body to an increase in external muscle load. These tests, such as the Shuttle Walk Test, the Step Test and the 6-Minute Test, do not seek to bring the individual up to his or her maximum load, but rather stop short of it. They are well-standardized tests that correlate well with oxygen consumption, the ability to perform activities of daily living and the tolerated load in laboratory exercise tests (20).

  - The 6-minute test: Consists of walking the maximum possible distance on level ground for 6 minutes, following a standardized protocol. This test has a good predictive value for mortality in COPD patients and is useful in those cases where performing a complete stress test is difficult. This test is characterized by its simplicity and low cost. The distance covered is an indicator of submaximal exercise tolerance capacity. These values constitute a severity marker independent of lung function measured by FEV1 and allow a rapid interpretation of the evolution of the disease, facilitating the clinical evaluation of the patient (29). To carry out this test, an adequate physical space is required, preferably a flat terrain of at least 30 meters in length, and the necessary equipment, which includes a pulse oximeter, a stopwatch, cones to mark the course, a Borg scale, and transportable oxygen if necessary, among others. The personnel in charge of administering these tests should have an appropriate qualification in nursing, physiotherapy or medicine, as well as skills in dealing with patients, knowledge of exercise physiology in the sick, decision-making skills and knowledge of cardiopulmonary resuscitation. It is important that patients are properly prepared for these tests, which includes wearing comfortable clothing and footwear, having a light meal, avoiding strenuous exercise beforehand, and adhering to the usual medication schedule. To ensure the reliability of the results, it is recommended to perform two tests and select the best one for interpretation. In addition, factors that may influence the results, such as height, age, overweight, patient motivation, and the effect of medication, among others, should be considered (29).

Prueba de seis minutos marcha - 6MWT　　Hoja 1

Nombre		Fecha

Sexo (H/M)	Edad (años)	Peso (Kg)	Talla (m)

Diagnóstico		Examinador

Medicación (incluir dosis y horario)

6MWT Nº1	30	metros			SaO2 (sentado, en reposo aire ambiente(%))
Valores basales					
SaO2		(%)			Oxigeno suplemt. (lpm)
FC		(ppm)			
Disnea		(Borg)			SaO2 (con oxigeno suplemt.(%))
Fatiga EEII		(Borg)			

Vueltas	Metros	Tiempo	SaO2	FC	Incentivo
1	30				
2	60				min 1 "Lo está haciendo muy bien, faltan 5 minutos"
3	90				
4	120				
5	150				min 2 "Perfecto, continúe así, faltan 4 minutos"
6	180				
7	210				
8	240				min 3 "Está en la mitad del tiempo de la prueba, lo está haciendo muy bien"
9	270				
10	300				
11	330				min 4 "Perfecto, continúe así, faltan dos minutos"
12	360				
13	390				
14	420				min 5 "Lo está haciendo muy bien, falta un minuto"
15	450				
16	480				
17	510				min 6 Quince segundos antes de finalizar: "deberá detenerse cuando se lo indique" Al minuto 6: "pare, la prueba ha finalizado"
18	540				
19	570				
20	600				

Valores finales 6MWT		
SaO2		(%)
FC		(ppm)
Disnea		(Borg)
Fatiga EEII		(Borg)
Distancia total caminada		(m)
Nº paradas		-
Tiempo total paradas		(min)

Observaciones

Figure 18. Documentation to be filled out for the six-minute walk test (29).

- The Incremental Shuttle Walk Test (ISWT): Performed over a distance of 10 meters with 12 speed levels, it aims to achieve the highest possible distance covered and walking speed level while maintaining the pace set by the test's acoustic signals. This test is well standardized and highly reproducible, comparable to laboratory tests. In addition, it is sensitive to pre-

and post-treatment changes and correlates with other parameters such as maximal oxygen consumption (VO2 peak), quality of life and other similar tests.

However, it has some limitations, such as the lack of additional information to the incremental stress test, the lack of established normality values, and the need for a sound player. In addition, it may be less accurate in determining elevated velocity levels and requires high motivation on the part of the patient. To carry out the test, it is performed in a flat corridor of at least 10 meters in length, delimited by cones. During the test, the patient walks back and forth following the acoustic signals indicating changes in speed level. It is important that the patient is properly briefed on how to perform the test before the test begins, including instructions on walking speed, cone placement, and how to respond if he or she feels unwell during the test. Vital signs and levels of dyspnea and fatigue are recorded before and after the test to assess the patient's response (29).

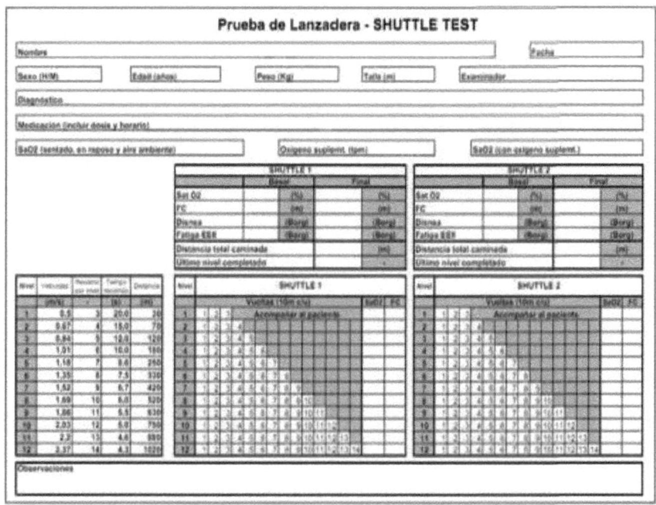

Figure 19. Shuttle test documentation (29).

- The Step Test, although less standardized, can be performed in two ways: by setting the number of steps the patient must go up and down in a given time, or by setting a time and evaluating how many steps the patient can go up and down in that time.
- Quality of life assessment:

The assessment of health-related quality of life (HRQoL) is crucial to understanding the impact of illness, injury, treatment or health policy on the lives of individuals and communities. It is used to assess how these aspects may affect people's lives in terms of well-being and functionality, as opposed to simply how long they live. There are questionnaires specifically designed to assess HRQoL, which look at physical activity limitation, emotional impact, social impact and symptoms. Dyspnea, due to its frequency and impact on daily activities, is one of the key symptoms assessed in these questionnaires (9). These questionnaires are divided into two main groups: generic and specific. The generic ones allow the health status of diverse populations to be assessed, while the specific ones focus on a particular disease and how it affects the individual. Examples of generic questionnaires include the Sickness Impact Profile, Nottingham Health Profile, SF-36 and Quality of Well-Being. For COPD, specific questionnaires are used such as the Chronic Respiratory Questionnaire (CRQ), St. George's Respiratory Questionnaire (SGRQ), Respiratory Quality of Life Questionnaire (RQLQ) and the COPD Assessment Test (CAT). The CAT, in particular, is a simple and reliable tool for measuring COPD-related health status. It is not a diagnostic test, but a way to assess quality of life. A difference of 2 points or more on the CAT is considered clinically significant, and can complement information obtained from other tests such as lung function (9).

COPD Assessment Test Questionnaire							
I never cough	0	1	2	3	4	5	I cough all the time
I have no phlegm (mucus in my chest).	0	1	2	3	4	5	I have a chest full of phlegm (mucus).
I don't feel my chest tight	0	1	2	3	4	5	My chest feels tight

I am not short of breath when climbing slopes or stairs.	0	1	2	3	4	5	I get short of breath when climbing slopes or stairs
I have no limitation for household chores	0	1	2	3	4	5	I am totally limited for household chores
I have no problem leaving my home	0	1	2	3	4	5	I don't feel safe to leave my home
I sleep soundly	0	1	2	3	4	5	My breathing problem prevents me from sleeping
I have a lot of energy	0	1	2	3	4	5	I don't have any energy

Questionnaire for COPD patient symptomatology: COPD Assessment Test (9).

- Assessment of physical activity:

Physical activity plays an important role in the progression and prognosis of COPD. During exacerbations of the disease, physical activity tends to decrease and this reduction is maintained even after recovery. Although respiratory rehabilitation can improve exercise tolerance, it does not always translate into a significant increase in physical activity levels in COPD patients.

A useful tool for assessing physical activity in the population is the International Physical Activity Questionnaire (IPAQ). This questionnaire is used to determine the amount of physical exercise performed by the population through a self-administered survey. There are two versions of the IPAQ: a short one, with 9 items that ask about time spent on different levels of activity and sedentary activities, and a long one, with 31 items that also include information on domestic, occupational, transportation and leisure activities, as well as sedentary activities.

3.3. Respiratory pathologies and physiotherapeutic intervention.

Lung diseases can be classified into two main categories: obstructive and restrictive.

- Obstructive Diseases: These conditions cause resistance to airflow in the airways. Examples of obstructive diseases include asthma, chronic obstructive pulmonary disease (COPD), bronchiectasis, emphysema, cystic fibrosis, among others.

- Restrictive Diseases: These diseases affect the pulmonary interstitium, reducing the ability of the lungs to expand and contract properly. Examples of restrictive diseases are sarcoidosis, pneumoconiosis, idiopathic pulmonary fibrosis, neuromuscular diseases, thoracic deformities, pleural effusion, pneumothorax, diaphragmatic paralysis or paresis, thoracotomy, among others.

The approach to physiotherapeutic treatment in these patients should be based on the individual characteristics of each patient and their clinical evaluation, rather than focusing solely on the diagnosis of a specific pathology. It is considered more appropriate to combine several techniques rather than applying a single standardized technique for all patients. However, for study purposes, the physiotherapeutic treatment can be simplified and described according to the pathology.

3.3.1. Pathologies with obstructive ventilatory alterations.
3.3.1.1. Bronchiolitis:

Bronchiolitis is a pathological process that is not specific to a single disease, but can be caused by several different conditions. It is characterized by inflammatory changes in the smaller airways, especially in the terminal bronchioles. This disorder can vary in its clinical picture and prognosis, and usually affects predominantly the small airways, although occasionally it may also involve the larger airways or lung parenchyma, depending on its underlying cause. Bronchiolitis can occur as a primary disease, as a result of viral infection or exposure to toxic inhalants, among other factors. It can also occur as part of a broader lung disease, such as hypersensitivity pneumonitis, chronic obstructive pulmonary disease (COPD), or connective tissue disorders such as collagenopathies. In both cases, the symptoms and course of the disease may vary depending on the underlying cause and severity of bronchiolar involvement (28).

Bronchiolitis can also present in pediatric age as a common disease in children under 2 years of age, predominantly between 2 and 10 months of age. The main agent is Respiratory Syncytial Virus (RSV). It initially affects the upper respiratory tract and then progresses to the lower respiratory tract within 48 to 72 hours. This leads to epithelial necrosis, cilia-free regeneration, mucosal edema and airway obstruction, increasing ventilatory work. Bronchial lesions may persist into adulthood. The classification of bronchiolitis is based on clinical criteria, such as the Wood-Downes scale modified by Ferrés for severity, and the Silverman scale for respiratory evaluation in neonates (30).

- Clinical manifestations are (30):
  - Wheezing.
  - Coughing.
  - Dyspnea.
  - Hyperinflation.
- Physiotherapy treatment: In mild and moderate cases, bronchial hygiene techniques are used, such as upper airway clearance, spontaneous or provoked cough, together with hypertonic saline, forced expiratory techniques, slow passive expiratory techniques and retrograde rhinopharyngeal clearance (30).

3.3.1.2. Cystic Fibrosis or Mucoviscidosis:

It is an autosomal recessive inherited disease that affects the exocrine glands, especially in the respiratory, digestive, skin and genital systems. The lungs are the most affected, presenting an increase in mucus production. The sweat test is useful for diagnosis, where elevated concentrations of sodium and chloride in sweat are indicative. Clinical manifestations include chronic sinusitis, persistent cough, thick sputum, periods of stability interrupted by exacerbations, among others (31).

- Physiotherapy treatment (31):
  - It is recommended to perform bronchial hygiene techniques, adapted according to the patient's age.
  - In infants, passive techniques such as prolonged slow expiration with tracheal pumping and induced coughing are used.
  - In older children, nasal lavage, drainage of bronchial secretions, assisted autogenous drainage, prolonged slow expiration,

increased expiratory flow with active participation of the patient are encouraged.

- In adults, nasal lavage, evacuation technique, drainage of bronchial secretions, slow total expiration with infralateral open glottis, autogenous drainage, oscillating and non-oscillating positive expiratory pressure (PEP) devices, ventilation and lung expansion exercises are performed.
- Devices such as discontinuous expiratory pressure devices can facilitate secretion drainage.
- Physical exercise and pulmonary rehabilitation are also beneficial to improve quality of life. The recommended weekly dose for children and adolescents will be at least 60 minutes of moderate-intensity physical activity on all or most days of the week, or vigorous intensity 3 days a week. While for adults a minimum of 150 minutes of moderate physical activity per week, or 75 minutes of vigorous physical activity should be performed.

3.3.1.3. Asthma:

The definition of asthma according to the Global Initiative for Asthma (G.I.N.A) is "chronic inflammation of the airways, in which certain cells and mediators play a prominent role" (32).

- Clinical manifestations:
  - Bronchial hyperreactivity leading to smooth muscle constriction, edema and excessive mucus production.
  - Exacerbations with recurrent episodes of wheezing, dyspnea, chest tightness, dry cough especially at night, among other symptoms.
  - X-rays may show thickened bronchial walls, hyperinflation and atelectasis in severe cases.
- Genetic and environmental components: Asthma has a genetic component and is associated with a family history of asthma, rhinitis, atopic eczema, and allergic disorders. It is also related to environmental, physical, infectious and occupational factors.
- Assessment and diagnosis:

- There are several scales to measure the severity of seizures, such as the Scarfone Score.
- Spirometry is a crucial adjunctive test that assesses bronchial patency.
- Peak expiratory flow (PEF) is also useful for monitoring clinical progress and can be used at the patient's home.
- Pharmacological treatment: In cases of severe bronchoconstriction, oxygen therapy, β-agonists bronchodilators and systemic corticosteroids are used. In addition, hyperosmolar aerosols may be administered to facilitate expectoration. An active combat against allergens and other predisposing factors is carried out.
- Physiotherapy Objectives and Treatment
  - Decrease hyperventilation.
  - Relax the accessory musculature.
  - Addressing respiratory blockages.
- Techniques (32):
  - During the intercrisis phase, breathing control is emphasized, with emphasis on awareness of the diaphragm and its role in ventilation. Diaphragmatic and lung expansion exercises are practiced and tidal volume, respiratory rate and ventilatory rate are monitored.
  - To alleviate anxiety and dyspnea, body positions that facilitate breathing, such as upright sitting or the tripod position, are adopted.
  - Massage therapy and spinal mobilizations promote optimal rib mobilization and relaxation of the inspiratory accessory musculature.
  - In case of bronchospasm, pursed-lip expiration is recommended, while directed coughing and forced expiration technique are discouraged.
  - Irritative cough inhibitory techniques are taught, such as the Valsalva maneuver and shallow breathing.
  - It is essential to keep the airway clear of secretions in patients with respiratory conditions. To achieve this, clearance techniques such as autogenous drainage, ELTGOL and positive expiratory

pressure techniques such as Flutter, Acapella and Thera PEP are used, which not only promote clearance of secretions, but also increase intrabronchial pressure, preventing airway collapse.

- Health education is an integral part of treatment, teaching proper inhalation technique and management of crisis episodes.
- Breathing exercises are important tools in the management of asthma, as they help control breathing and can reduce symptoms. Some of the most commonly used exercises in patients with asthma are (32):
  - Buteyko Technique: This technique focuses on nasal breathing to control ventilation. It is characterized by breathing through the nose and through ventilatory pauses to increase alveolar and arterial carbon dioxide (CO_2) tension. The goal is to reduce bronchospasm, normalize the breathing pattern and reduce the sensation of dyspnea.
  - Diaphragmatic Respiratory Re-education (DRR): This technique aims at recovering the diaphragmatic ventilatory pattern, which is essential for proper breathing. It is combined with slow nasal breathing and lengthening of the exhalation to improve respiratory control.
  - Papworth Method: Consists of using a diaphragmatic breathing pattern along with relaxation techniques and education to reduce hyperventilation and hyperinflation. It increases CO_2 levels and decreases the effects of hypocapnia, as well as symptoms related to bronchospasm.
  - Pranayama breathing: This is the breathing technique used in yoga. It is characterized by deep breaths with the diaphragm and a slow breathing rate, using the nose. This technique can help improve respiratory control and reduce anxiety associated with dyspnea in patients with asthma.

3.3.1.4. Bronchiectasis:

Bronchiectasis is characterized by the abnormal, permanent and irreversible dilatation of one or more bronchi due to chronic inflammation of their wall. This leads to the destruction of the elastic, muscular and cartilaginous component, together with the loss of cilia, resulting in the production of mucopurulent secretions. Bronchiectasis is usually the final consequence of various pathologies that injure the bronchial tree, with infection being the common cause. They can be classified as cylindrical (less wall destruction), cystic (great wall destruction) and varicose (intermediate destruction), being more common in women (23).

- Clinical manifestations:
  - Acropaquias.
  - Roncus.
  - Wheezing.
  - Coughing.
  - Daily expectoration with mucopurulent secretions.
  - Dyspnea.
  - Variable hemoptysis associated with exacerbations.
  - Fever.
  - Chest pain.
  - Symptoms of rhinosinusitis.
  - In advanced stages: malnutrition and generalized deterioration of health status.

During functional assessment, spirometry may reveal a normal or obstructive pattern. Bronchiectasis is most often located in the lung bases, middle lobe and lingula. On blood gases, hypoxemia and hypercapnia are commonly observed.

- Physiotherapeutic modalities used in the management of bronchiectasis (23):
  - Therapeutic Aerosols:
    - Ultrasonic nebulization of isotonic saline solution: Consists of the inhalation of a saline solution using an ultrasonic nebulizer. It helps to moisten the airways and facilitate the elimination of secretions.

- N-acetyl-L-cysteine: This mucolytic is used to reduce the viscosity of bronchial secretions, facilitating their expulsion and improving respiratory function.
- Bronchial Hygiene Techniques:
  - Institutional: Postural drainage, assisted cough maneuvers, expiratory flow acceleration.
  - Domiciliary: Autogenous drainage, Eltgol, positive expiratory pressure techniques (Thera PEP, Flutter, Cornet, Acapella).

3.3.1.5. Chronic Obstructive Pulmonary Disease (COPD)

Chronic Obstructive Lung Disease (COPD) is defined by the Global Initiative for Chronic Obstructive Lung Disease (GOLD) as a treatable and preventable condition characterized by the persistent presence of respiratory symptoms and airflow limitation due to changes in the alveoli and/or airways, generally caused by prolonged exposure to noxious substances such as gases or particles. The Spanish GesEPOC guide describes the disease as a reversible chronic airflow limitation mainly associated with tobacco smoke. According to the Spanish Society of Pneumology and Thoracic Surgery (SEPAR), COPD is characterized by a chronic, poorly reversible airflow obstruction, mainly caused by an abnormal inflammatory response to tobacco smoke (33).

The clinical diagnosis is established by airflow limitation and is classified into four degrees of severity according to the FEV1 value. In addition, a new assessment method called "ABCD" has been incorporated, which is not only based on the severity of airflow obstruction (FEV1), but also considers patient perception, dyspnea and quality of life. Quality of life is a crucial aspect highlighted, along with the importance of history of exacerbations. Dyspnea is assessed using the Modified Medical Research Council (mMRC) scale, while quality of life is determined by the COPD Assessment Test (CAT) questionnaire. Currently, the GOLD classification to determine the severity of COPD considers mainly three factors: the intensity of symptoms, the degree of airflow limitation (FEV1) and the history of exacerbations (33).

The clinical presentation of COPD is highly variable, and within what is currently known as COPD, there are different clinical forms or phenotypes that have clinical, prognostic and therapeutic implications.

- These phenotypes include:
    - Non-exacerbating, with emphysema or chronic bronchitis.
    - Mixed COPD-Asthma.
    - Acute with emphysema
    - Exacerbator with chronic bronchitis.
- Characteristics of COPD:
    - Dyspnea: Usually experienced during daily activities, especially when using the upper limbs.
    - Coughing.
    - Expectoration.
    - Wheezing.
    - Systemic symptoms such as anorexia and peripheral muscle involvement.
    - Radiographs show rib horizontalization and flattened diaphragmatic domes.
    - Spirometry: There is evidence of an increase in residual volume and total lung capacity, accompanied by a decrease in vital capacity.
- Some physiotherapeutic modalities used to reduce airflow obstruction in COPD patients (33):
    - Management of bronchospasm: Anticholinergic sprays are very useful in the treatment of bronchospasm in COPD patients, as they help to reduce the increased cholinergic tone in these patients. In addition to anticholinergics, inhaled beta-adrenergics are also administered for the management of bronchospasm.

    - Management of bronchial lumen occupancy:
        - Bronchial wall edema: The management of bronchial edema is a medical competence, and may include the use of corticosteroids.

- - - Mucosal gland hypertrophy: Glandular hypertrophy corresponds to irreversible structural damage. Smoking cessation is essential for the management of this condition.
    - Increase of secretions: To reduce or eliminate bronchial occupation by secretions, therapeutic sprays with humectant, mucokinetic or mucolytic qualities are used. In addition, bronchial hygiene techniques are used to mobilize and eliminate secretions.
  - Management of loss of radial traction on the bronchus: In patients with pulmonary emphysema, loss of radial traction on the bronchus is an important cause of airflow obstruction. Physiotherapeutic techniques, such as maximal inspiration followed by active expiration with abdominal muscle intervention, can be used to maximize bronchial opening and facilitate removal of trapped air.
- Physiotherapeutic modalities used to improve respiratory muscle function in patients with COPD (23):
  - Respiratory reeducation: This strategy aims at recovering the physiological respiratory pattern, normalizing the tidal volume, reducing the respiratory frequency and maintaining an adequate relation between inspiration and expiration. The aim is to improve the efficiency of respiratory muscle function, reverse as far as possible the alterations in the ventilation/perfusion (V/Q) ratio, improve mobility and flexibility of the rib cage, and increase tolerance to daily activities.
  - Respiratory re-education techniques: Diaphragmatic breathing, pursed-lip breathing, non-specific breathing exercises: These exercises are designed to improve the mobility and flexibility of the rib cage, which facilitates more efficient breathing.
  - Thoracic mobilizations: These techniques involve physical manipulations aimed at improving the mobility of the thoracic joints and structures, which can facilitate more complete and effective breathing.
  - Targeted ventilation: This technique focuses on practicing specific breathing patterns to improve ventilation in specific

areas of the lungs. It may include deep breathing exercises and chest expansion techniques.

Patients with COPD may present with emphysema or chronic bronchitis (23).

- Emphysema:

Emphysema is characterized by dilatation of the air spaces distal to the terminal bronchiole, accompanied by destruction of the alveolar walls. This leads to poor gas exchange between the alveoli (due to their reduced number) and the blood circulation. There are three main types of emphysema:

- Centroacinar or centrolobulillar: It mainly affects the central part of the pulmonary lobule, without significantly altering the alveoli, their vascularization or their peripheral ducts. It is usually located at the apex of the upper lobe.
- Panacinar or panlobulillar: It causes the destruction and distension of the entire lobule or acinus, affecting both the peripheral alveoli and their vascularization. It is more common in the lower lobes or bases and is associated with alpha-1 antitrypsin deficiency, being a primary autoimmune disease with no history of smoking.
- Paraseptal or distal: It affects the lobular periphery, close to the pleura, and is located in the intralobular areas. Sometimes it does not affect pulmonary ventilation significantly.
- Clinical manifestations of emphysema include:
    - Physical appearance of "pink puffer" or "pink puffer".
    - Thin constitution.
    - Barrel-shaped thorax due to increased anteroposterior diameter.
    - Intense progressive dyspnea.
    - Intercostal retractions, reduced diaphragmatic breathing and hypertrophy of accessory muscles of respiration.
    - Moderately low oxygen levels at rest (PaO2 between 60 mmHg) and normal or slightly elevated carbon dioxide levels.

- - - Possibility of congestive heart failure.
    - Cough with white expectoration without cyanosis.
    - X-rays may show descended diaphragms, excessive pulmonary distension, shortening of diaphragmatic muscle fibers, horizontal ribs, bulla formation (thin-walled subpleural air spaces), vascular rarefaction and narrowing of peripheral pulmonary vessels.
    - Spirometry shows an increase in residual volume and total lung capacity, accompanied by a decrease in vital capacity.
- Chronic bronchitis is an obstructive disease of the peripheral airways that develops due to tobacco use, recurrent infections, exposure to environmental pollution and allergies. It is characterized by excessive mucus production in the airways, caused by hypertrophy of the mucous glands of the trachea and bronchi, which can obstruct the airways and smaller bronchioles. In addition, stenosis of the airways and edema in their walls are observed. It is considered chronic when there is productive, irritative cough and expectoration for at least 3 months per year, for a period of at least 2 consecutive years, excluding other causes of productive cough. Clinical manifestations of chronic bronchitis include:
  - Physical appearance known as "bluish congestive" or "blue bloater".
  - Pronounced cyanosis.
  - Obese constitution.
  - Prevalence in smokers.
  - Moderate dyspnea progressing to exertional dyspnea.
  - Low oxygen and high carbon dioxide levels in the blood.
  - Chronic cough.
  - Auscultation with scattered crackles and rhonchi.
  - Normal or slightly increased thoracic volume, with hypersonority to percussion and possible peripheral edema.
  - On radiographs, signs such as slight cardiomegaly, congested lung areas, enlarged vascular network and swollen bronchi may be seen. Over time, a "dirty lung" may be seen due to thickening of the bronchial walls and peribronchial fibrosis.

These symptoms may improve if the causes that led to the bronchitis are eliminated. In addition, chronic bronchitis may coexist with emphysema.

3.3.2. Pathologies with restrictive ventilatory alterations

3.3.2.1. Pneumonia

Pneumonia is an inflammation of the lung parenchyma, which is located distal to the terminal bronchi, and is infectious in origin. The causative agents of pneumonia vary according to the location where they are acquired, the age of the individual and the presence of underlying diseases. In children, viral pneumonias are common, while in adults those of bacterial origin predominate. Clinically, it is characterized by fever, variable respiratory symptoms and an infiltrate on chest X-ray. It develops due to the presence of a pathogen together with a dysfunction in the pulmonary defense mechanisms. Depending on where the infection originates, it is classified into (34):

- Community-acquired pneumonia (CAP): Occurs in people who have not been recently hospitalized.
- Nosocomial pneumonia: Occurs within 48 hours after hospitalization, generally associated with prolonged hospital stays and invasive airway procedures. It is usually caused by methicillin-resistant Staphylococcus Aureus.

Physiotherapy treatment: During the acute phase of the disease, respiratory physiotherapy is contraindicated. Once the fever has progressively decreased, lung expansion techniques are performed and functional exercises are completed.

- Physiotherapeutic treatment (34):
    - To increase exhaled volume Mobilization/Positioning we use breathing exercises, incentive spirometry and manual or mechanical hyperinflation.
    - To increase Expiratory Flow Positioning: Huff, Manual Assisted Cough, Mechanical Cough Assist, Percussive Oscillation, Mechanical or Manual Vibration, HFO, IPV, Flutter
    - Increase Exhaled Volume Positioning: CPAP and PEP

3.3.2.2. Diffuse Interstitial Lung Disease (DIDD)

Diffuse fibrosing alveolitis, also known as diffuse interstitial lung disease (DIDP), diffuse interstitial pulmonary fibrosis or Hamman-Rich syndrome, affects the alveolar-interstitial space with clinical, functional and radiological manifestations. Among DIDF, the most common are idiopathic pulmonary fibrosis and sarcoidosis. Clinical manifestations include exertional dyspnea and dry cough, diffuse bilateral infiltrates, restrictive functional alterations and decreased diffusion. Pulmonary fibrosis is a specific form of DIDP, characterized as a diffuse, fibrosing, chronic, progressive, interstitial lung disease, mainly affecting older men. The characteristic radiological pattern is "honeycombing", consisting of clusters of cystic airspaces of comparable diameters of 3-10 mm (sometimes up to 2.5 cm). Possible risk factors include smoking, exposure to metal or wood dust, agricultural activities, work in hairdressing, stone cutting or polishing, exposure to livestock and plant or animal dusts, as well as chemotherapy, although with little evidence (9).

Physiotherapy goals and treatment: The goals of treatment are to improve ventilatory dynamics, reduce the risk of infections, prevent thoracic deformities and improve exercise tolerance. In terms of respiratory physiotherapy treatment, lung expansion techniques such as Inspiratory Diameter Costal Exercise (EDIC), costal expansion techniques, diaphragmatic and spinal exercises, among others, can help alleviate symptoms. In advanced stages, lung transplantation may be considered. Respiratory rehabilitation is safe in patients with IDPD and improves quality of life (9).

3.3.2.3. Pulmonary Abscess

A lung abscess is a suppurative collection that forms as a result of necrosis of the lung parenchyma, resulting in the creation of a cavity with its own walls. Clinical manifestations include dyspnea, productive cough, foul-smelling and copious expectoration, pleuritic pain, nausea, vomiting, chills, sweating and malaise. In some cases, acropacities may appear (19).

It is true that the use of physiotherapy and postural drainage in the acute phase in the treatment of lung abscess may be controversial due to the potential risk of spread of infection. It has been observed that the manipulation of secretions and the application of physiotherapy techniques may contribute to the spread of infection in the respiratory tract. In the specific case of lung abscess, thoracic drainage is mainly reserved for cases of empyema, where there is accumulation of pus in the pleural cavity. However, nowadays, due to the efficacy of antimicrobials, it is not common to indicate transthoracic drainage of the abscess or its surgical resection, unless there are severe complications or medical treatment is ineffective. It is important to carefully evaluate each individual case and consider the risks and benefits of physical therapy and other interventions, always in coordination with the treating medical team. The therapeutic approach may vary depending on the severity of the infection, the response to antimicrobial treatment and the presence of additional complications (19).

- Medical treatment may involve the use of chemotherapy, bronchoaspiration or segmental excision to remove the abscess.
- Physical therapy treatment:
    - Once the abscess has been drained, the goal of physical therapy treatment is to achieve re-expansion of the affected area. This can be achieved by:
    - Postural drainage to facilitate drainage of secretions.
    - Localized ventilation exercises, focusing on exhalation to help eliminate secretions.
    - Assisted cough to clear the airway.
    - Complement treatment with aerosol therapy using antibiotics to treat pulmonary infection.
- This approach to respiratory physiotherapy helps improve ventilation and promote patient recovery after medical treatment for lung abscess.

3.3.2.4. Pleural effusion

It is the accumulation of fluid in the pleural space, partially or totally, due to an imbalance between the formation and reabsorption of this fluid. According to its characteristics, it can be (19):

- Transudate: fluid poor in proteins and cells, resulting from an increase in hydrostatic pressure and a reduction in the oncotic pressure of the pleural capillaries.
- Exudate: fluid rich in proteins and cells, caused by increased permeability of capillaries or lymphatic obstruction. It may present as serofibrinous, purulent (empyema or pyrothorax), hemorrhagic (hemothorax) or lymphatic (chylothorax).

In the presence of an inflammatory process, pleural flanges may form. In cases of purulent pleuritis, sclerosis and encystation may develop. In the case of hemothorax, blood tends to coagulate early (19).

- Clinical manifestations:
  - Dyspnea.
  - Pleuritic pain.
  - Dry cough.
  - Hypomobility of the affected hemithorax.
  - Deviation of the mediastinum towards the healthy side.
  - Adhesions on the affected side limiting the respiratory pattern and mobility of the hemidiaphragm.
  - Dull sound to percussion. In the case of pneumothorax, the sound will be tympanic.
  - Patients tend to lie in lateral decubitus on the affected side or semi-sitting position to minimize pain.
- Physiotherapy objectives and treatment:
  - Avoid the formation of adhesions.
  - Reexpand the lung parenchyma.
  - To prevent alterations in respiratory mechanics.
  - Eliminate secretions in case of accumulation.

Physiotherapeutic treatment involves thoracic mobilization of the affected side, hemidiaphragm work and thoracic cage flexibilization with corrective exercises of the spine and shoulder girdle. The treatment sequence may include (19):

- Early phase: Slow and deep diaphragmatic respirations, combined with analgesic treatment.
- Second phase: Lung expansion techniques.
- Third phase: Intensification of lung expansion techniques.

For recurrent or poorly managed pleural disease, diaphragmatic pattern techniques can be used, with the patient in lateral decubitus on the affected side.

3.3.2.5. Pneumothorax

Pneumothorax is caused by air entering the pleural space, which causes the lung to collapse and hinders its expansion. This results in distension of the rib cage and depression of the affected hemidiaphragm, which in turn reduces FEV1 (forced expiratory volume in the first second) and FVC (forced vital capacity) (35).

- Types of pneumothorax (35).
    - Spontaneous: occurs from rupture of a bulla at the apex of the lung, often associated with diseases such as COPD. Symptoms include sudden pain, dyspnea and decreased breath sounds on the affected side.
    - Traumatic:
    - Closed: visceral pleural injury with intact chest wall.
    - Open: opening of the chest wall that allows atmospheric air to enter the pleural space.
    - Tension: rupture that creates a unidirectional valve, increasing the pressure in the pleural space. Requires urgent medical intervention.
    - Iatrogenic: secondary to medical procedures.
- Assessment: Galliard's triad may be found on physical examination:
    - Tympanic sound in thoracic percussion.
    - Decreased vocal vibrations.
    - Decreased vesicular murmur.
- Physiotherapy objectives and treatment (35):

- Assist lung expansion, provided there is drainage.
- Avoid adhesion formation and maintain diaphragmatic mobility.
- Physiotherapeutic treatment involves placing the patient in lateral decubitus on the healthy side, alternating with anterior and posterior rotation. Drains are monitored and global ventilation exercises are performed, focusing on prolonged expiration. Once the drains are removed, ventilation exercises adapted to activities of daily living are continued.

3.3.2.6. Neuromuscular Diseases (NMD)

Neuromuscular diseases (NMDs) comprise a diverse group of neurological disorders caused by primary or secondary alterations in musculoskeletal cells. In most of these disorders, progressive deterioration of muscles, including respiratory muscles, is observed, which can lead to weakness (36).

- Clinical manifestations: Clinical manifestations vary according to the degree of involvement of the patient's respiratory muscles, swallowing muscles and mobility ability. Although the lung is usually normal, the chest wall may be weak. Respiratory muscle involvement may result in a restrictive pattern, with reduced tidal volume and inspiratory capacity, making alveolar ventilation difficult. Ineffective cough and difficulty clearing secretions may arise from involvement of the expiratory musculature, increasing the risk of respiratory infections. The involvement of the oropharyngeal musculature can lead to problems in the swallowing mechanism and increase the risk of bronchoaspiration (36).
- Physical therapy treatment: Physical therapy treatment for patients with ENM focuses on maintaining lung compliance and rib cage mobility. Bronchial hygiene techniques are used and coughing is facilitated, either by manual assistance or with mechanical insufflation/exsufflation devices. The aim is to prevent respiratory complications and maintain pulmonary function as far as possible (36).

3.3.2.7. Atelectasis

Atelectasis is characterized by the total or partial collapse of part of the lung due to the disappearance of air contents, caused by airway obstruction, external pressure on the lung or surfactant dysfunction (23).

- Clinical manifestations (23):
    - Difficulty in the expansion of the affected hemithorax.
    - Coughing.
    - In mild cases, it may be asymptomatic.
    - X-ray shows narrowing of the intercostal spaces due to volume loss, with retraction of adjacent structures.
    - Total absence of vesicular murmur.
    - The most common atelectasis occurs in the basal lobes.
- Risk factors:
    - Administration of anesthesia.
    - Use of breathing tubes.
    - Foreign body in the respiratory tract (more common in children).
    - Pulmonary diseases.
    - Pleural effusion.
    - Obstruction by mucus in the respiratory tract.
    - Shallow breathing, which may be caused by pain.
    - Prolonged bed rest with little change of position.
    - Tumors that obstruct the airways.
- Physiotherapy objectives and treatment: The main objective of respiratory physiotherapy is to restore ventilatory mechanics as soon as possible. To achieve this, respiratory exercises focused on the collapsed area are performed, using slow and prolonged inspiration techniques such as EDIC, together with frequent postural changes (23).

3.3.2.8. Pneumonectomy / Lobectomy

Pneumonectomy involves the total removal of a lung, while lobectomy involves the removal of a specific lung lobe (23).

- Physiotherapy objectives and treatment (23):
  - Pneumonectomy: After pneumonectomy, the goals of physical therapy include ensuring airway patency in case of secretions, maintaining ventilation on the healthy side and avoiding postures that may be harmful. Therefore, the patient should not be placed in lateral decubitus on the healthy side to avoid compression of the mediastinum. Instead, it is recommended that he/she should lie on the incorporated bed, and important measures should be taken to control pain.
  - Lobectomy: After a partial lobectomy, the physical therapy program should be adapted considering the surgical intervention and the patient's previous respiratory pathology. It will focus on the re-expansion of the rest of the lung and on correcting the ventilatory compensations of the healthy hemithorax. This is achieved with abdomino-diaphragmatic and rib cage expansion exercises, thus helping to improve respiratory function and prevent complications.

4. <u>TECHNIQUES AND MODALITIES OF TREATMENT IN RESPIRATORY PHYSIOTHERAPY</u>

There are two main categories to classify manual respiratory physiotherapy techniques. According to the Lyon Consensus Conference in 1994, these techniques are classified on the basis of two criteria (37).

- The physical-mechanical effect they produce, such as gravity, shock waves and gas compression.
- The therapeutic objectives they pursue.

They are classified according to (37):

- The location of the respiratory disorder, either in the extrathoracic or intra-thoracic airways.
- The type of breathing pattern used, such as slow or forced inspiratory breathing, and slow or forced expiratory breathing.

4.1. Secretion drainage techniques.

4.1.1. Techniques based on the action of gravity.

Techniques based on the action of gravity are fundamental in respiratory physiotherapy. One of them is postural drainage, which takes advantage of the vertical position of the bronchial tubes to facilitate the evacuation of pulmonary secretions through the force of gravity. This technique is applied by placing the patient in different specific positions. It is considered most effective when secretions are fluid and abundant, and is especially recommended for severe patients subjected to prolonged periods of bed rest (4).

- Various postures are used to drain different lung segments (4):
  - Superior lobe:
    - Apical segment: Sitting with a pillow behind the shoulder corresponding to the segment to be drained.
    - Anterior segment: Supine decubitus with knees bent and a pillow under the corresponding shoulder.
    - Posterior segment: Fowler's position, semi-sitting with the body slightly inclined backwards.

- Medial lobe (right) and lingula (left): Lateral decubitus with a pillow under the shoulder to be drained, knees flexed and the foot of the bed elevated.
- Inferior lobe:
    - Apical segment (Nelson or segment 6): Prone with a pillow under the hips.
    - Anterior segment: Supine decubitus with the foot of the bed elevated and a pillow under the shoulder of the segment to be drained.
    - Lateral segment: lateral decubitus with a pillow under the side and the foot of the bed elevated.
    - Posterior segment: prone with a pillow under the hips and the foot of the bed elevated.

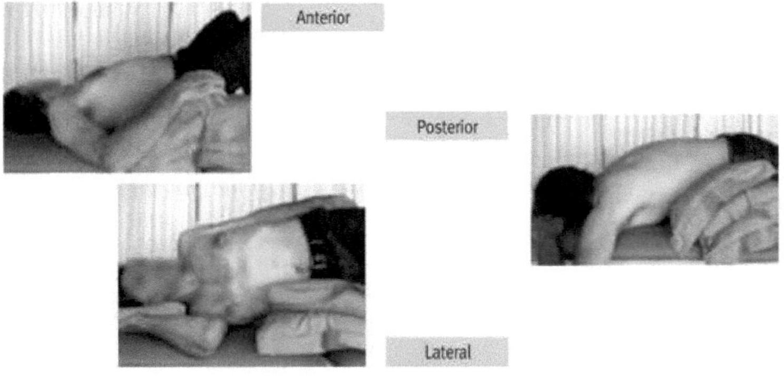

Figure 20. Postural drainage positions according to the pulmonary region to be treated (4).

It is important to note that these postures may vary depending on the pulmonary segment to be treated and the specific needs of the patient. In addition, there are contraindications for the use of postural drainage, such as bleeding, severe pulmonary edema, congestive heart failure, among others. It is essential to carefully evaluate each case before applying this technique.

4.1.2. Techniques based on shock waves.

Shockwave-based techniques are part of the assisted techniques and include manual vibrations and percussions, also known as clapping.

- Vibration: Vibration involves intermittent, rhythmic, progressive oscillatory movements applied to the chest wall perpendicular to the lung segments, with an ideal frequency of 13 Hz. Its objective is to stimulate cilia movement to increase the mobilization of secretions. This effect includes the modification of mucus viscosity and elasticity, being especially useful in pathologies with dense and adherent secretions (4).
    - Indications: Recommended in pathologies with highly viscous and adherent secretions.
    - Contraindications: Osteoporosis, bullous emphysema, recent thoracic surgery, pneumothorax, rib fractures, thoracic instability.
    - Vibrations can be manual, transmitted by the physiotherapist through the arm, or mechanical, applied by means of external or internal devices. Endogenous vibrations are performed with vibrating vests, while exogenous vibrations are applied with PEP devices, which will be described in the section on instrumental devices.

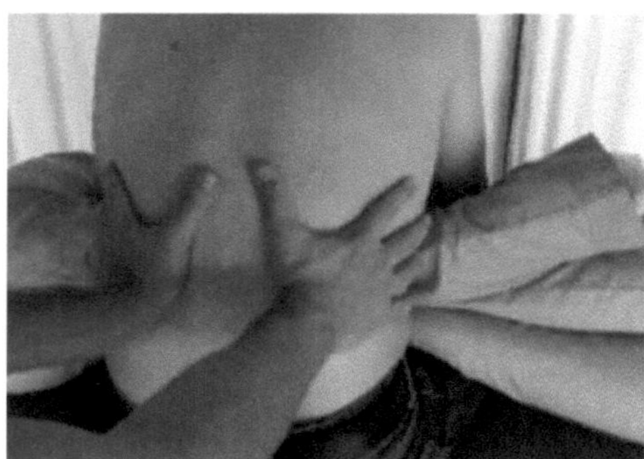

Figure 21. Vibration technique exerted on the base of the lungs with the patient seated (4).

- Percussions or clapping: Percussions consist of energetic and rhythmic tapping on the rib cage, using the hand in the form of a dome and performing flexion and extension movements of the wrist. The evidence on its efficacy is controversial (4).

- Contraindications: Bleeding pulmonary processes, thoracic surgery, pneumothorax, pleural effusion, emphysematous bullae, rib fractures, tuberculosis, pulmonary abscess, pulmonary neoplasia, bronchospasm, osteoporosis, among others.

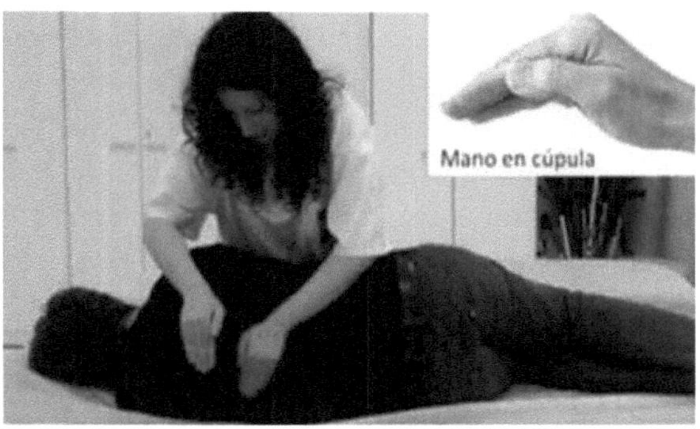

Figure 22. Application of the Clapping technique in the infralateral lung (4).

4.1.3. Techniques based on flow variations.

Techniques based on airflow variations focus on regulating and modulating expiratory flow. Four obstructive disorders in children (OBD) are identified, the first three (OBD I, II, III) being caused by excess secretions, while the fourth (OBD IV) results from the combination of secretions and bronchospasm. Depending on the location of the disorder, if it affects the extrathoracic airways, it is referred to as Obstructive Ventilatory Disorder I. This is diagnosed by direct auscultation or with phonendoscope, detecting noises transmitted by the excess of secretions. Treatment can be passive, by Retrograde Rhinopharyngeal Clearance (RRD), or active, such as nasoaspiration and nasal washes, especially in children, where nasal hygiene is essential to prevent contamination of the lower airways (37).

If the disorder affects the proximal intrathoracic airways, it is classified as Obstructive Ventilatory Disorder II, detectable by low frequency crackles on auscultation. This is treated with forced expiratory techniques. Finally, if the disorder affects the middle (5th-14th generation) or distal (16th-23rd generation) airways, it is termed Obstructive Ventilatory Disorder III, where medium and high frequency crackles are detected on auscultation. Treatment involves the use of slow expiratory techniques or techniques that generate volume-dependent effects, favoring pulmonary insufflation during inspiration (37).

4.1.3.1. Extrathoracic airways: Forced inspiratory techniques.

- Retrograde Rhinopharyngeal Clearance (RRD): RRD is a forced inspiratory technique designed to clear secretions from the nose and throat, often combined with the local application of a therapeutic substance. It is performed in children younger than 24 months; in older children, it can be performed by active nasoaspiration. The procedure is performed with the child lying on its back, with the head turned towards the side of the nostril to be cleaned. It consists of closing the child's mouth and, after provoking crying in most cases, inducing a sudden nasal inspiration while introducing saline at high pressure. The rapid inspiration following the crying serves as a vehicle for the saline (30).

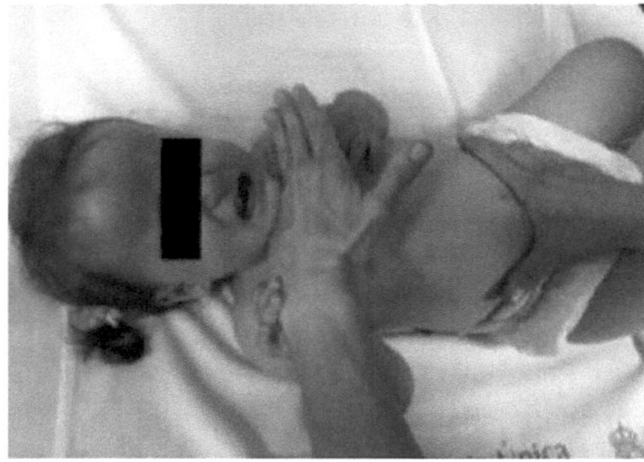

Figure 23. Retrograde rhinopharyngeal clearance technique. The dorsum of the hand resting on the maxilla to force the mouth to close (30).

- Retrograde glossopulsion (RGP): This technique involves guiding phlegm expelled by coughing from the back of the mouth to the lips, where it can be eliminated. It is used when the infant has difficulty expectorating (9).

- Expiratory Tracheal Pumping (ETP): Consists of placing the child in the supine position with the neck slightly extended backwards. This maneuver is performed by sliding the thumb along the extrathoracic trachea to drag the secretions upwards and facilitate their elimination (9).

4.1.3.2. Distal or middle intrathoracic airways: Slow expiratory techniques.

- Prolonged slow expiration (PrSLE): ELPr is a passive technique that aids in the expulsion of bronchial secretions from the middle airways to the proximal airways. It consists of applying joint manual pressure on the abdomen and thorax at the end of expiration up to the residual volume (RV). This pressure is gradual and is opposed to 2 or 3 inspiratory attempts (9).
- Lateral open glottic slow total expiration (ELTGOL): This technique is used to clear middle airway secretions. The patient is placed in lateral decubitus with the lung to be treated downward and is asked to perform a slow and prolonged open-glottic exhalation, starting from functional residual capacity (FRC) and maintaining low lung volumes. It is not suitable for infants and children under 10 or 12 years of age and is contraindicated in certain conditions such as hemoptysis, hemodynamic instability and cavitary conditions.

    Proper positioning of the physical therapist and patient to perform the thoracic percussion and vibration technique (ELTGOL) involves the physical therapist assisting the exhalation of the lung on the lower side by reducing the width of the thorax with his position on top of the patient's head, and by indirectly moving the diaphragm with his position on the lower side by performing rotational movements of the patient's forearm (4).

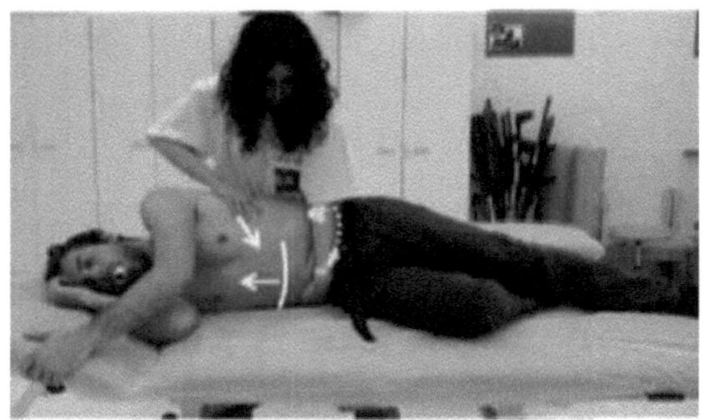

Figure 24. Correct position of the physiotherapist in the ETGOL technique (4).

- Autogenous drainage (AD): This technique, developed by Chevaillier in 1967, involves slow inhalations and exhalations to mobilize secretions. The patient is preferably seated with a straight back to optimize the interaction between the expiratory flow and the mucus surface. Autogenous Drainage is divided into four phases (4):
  - Phase 1. Clearance of secretions: During this phase, ventilation is performed at low lung volume to clear distal secretions. The patient's functional tidal volume moves within the expiratory reserve volume (ERV).
  - Phase 2. Accumulate or collect secretions: In this stage, ventilation is performed at half lung volume for the purpose of collecting secretions in the middle airways. The functional tidal volume shifts from the expiratory reserve volume (ERV) to the inspiratory reserve volume (IRV).
  - Phase 3. Evacuate secretions: During this phase, ventilation at medium or high volume is performed, starting from the middle of the LRV. This step is intended to facilitate the removal of accumulated secretions from the airway.
  - Final phase: After completing the three previous phases, a spontaneous cough may be induced or a forced expiratory technique (FET) may be used to remove any proximal secretions that may remain after the autogenous drainage process.

It is useful in diseases such as cystic fibrosis and bronchiectasis, but is contraindicated in asthma during acute crises.

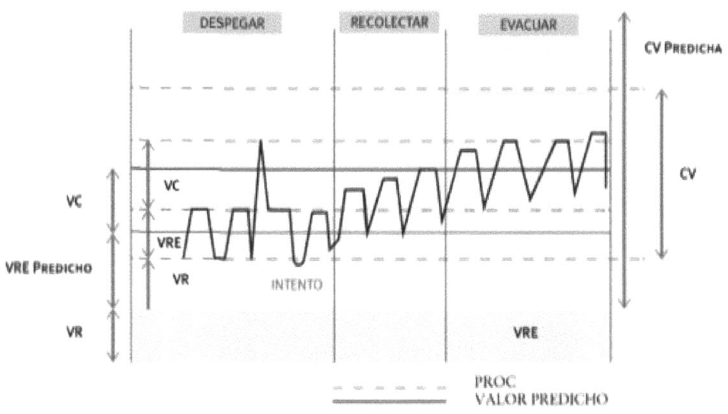

Figure 25. Representative diagram of the phases in autogenous drainage (4).

- Slow expiratory flow augmentation (slow EFA): This technique is used when secretions are in the middle or distal intrathoracic airways. After a moderate inspiration, expiratory flow is increased by a slow and prolonged exhalation, without forcing it. The physiotherapist can apply synchronized pressure in the thoracoabdominal region to increase the exhaled volume (9).

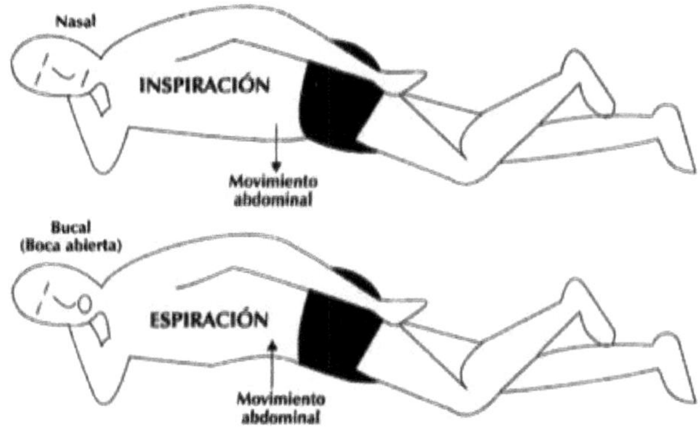

4.1.3.3. Proximal intrathoracic airways: Forced expiratory techniques

- Increased fast expiratory flow (AFE fast): After a wide inspiration, forced expiration with open glottis is performed. This technique may increase the tendency to airway closure and bronchospasm (9).
- Forced expiratory technique (FET): It is achieved after a wide inspiration by forceful contraction of the expiratory muscles. It is also included in the active respiratory cycle technique (4).

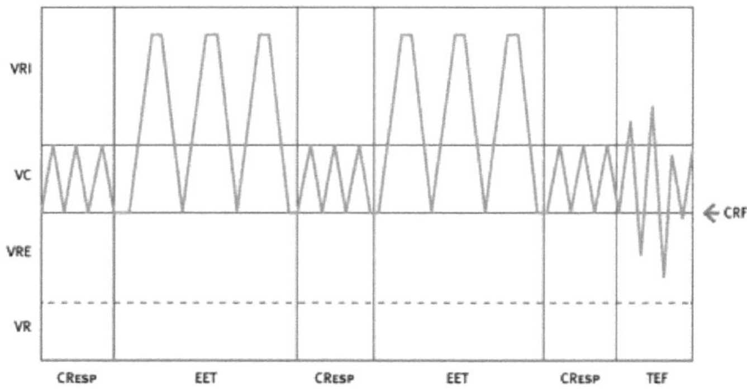

Figure 27. Lung volumes during the active respiratory cycle and forced expiratory technique (4).

- Active Cycling Respiratory Cycle (CAR) Technique: Seeks to mobilize and expel secretions from the middle and proximal airways. It is generally performed in a seated position, although it can also be done in other positions. It consists of a cycle of respiratory control, thoracic expansion and EFT. It is performed from a sequence of actions:
  - Respiratory control (slow and controlled diaphragmatic breathing) (4).
  - Thoracic expansion.
  - Respiratory control.
  - Thoracic expansion.
  - Respiratory control.

- TEF.
- Cough (T) (provoked, directed, assisted or spontaneous): It is used to dislodge and expel bronchial secretions in proximal airways. There is a sequence of essential phases in the cough maneuver for it to be effective and efficient (4):
    - Inspiratory phase: During this phase, there is abduction of the glottis and contraction of the diaphragm, along with some inspiratory accessory muscles, resulting in an increase in the elastic retraction pressure of the lung.
    - Compressive phase: In this stage, glottis adduction is combined with expiratory muscle contraction for approximately 0.2 seconds, which generates an increase in positive intrathoracic pressure.
    - Expiratory phase: During this phase, the air is rapidly expelled outwards thanks to the sudden opening of the glottis and the contraction of the expiratory muscles.

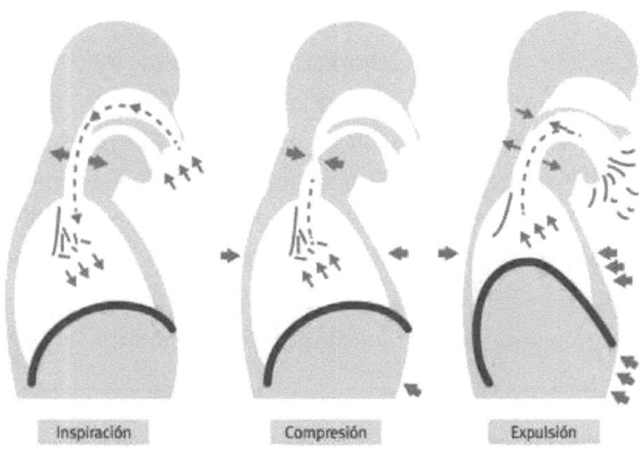

Figure 28. Phases of cough (4).

Effective and efficient cough maneuvering requires following a sequence of essential phases (4):
    - Provoked cough (PT): Induced by pressure on the sternal notch at the end of inspiration or beginning of expiration. It is

contraindicated in cases of vomiting reflex, laryngeal disorders and in premature newborns.

- Targeted cough (TD): It is a voluntary cough assisted by manual abdominal pressure. It is used in cooperative patients with secretions in proximal airways and trachea.
- Assisted cough: It is applied in cases of ineffective cough due to various causes, such as post-surgery pain or decreased expiratory flow due to secretions. It can be manual or by means of mechanical devices.

4.2. Costal expansion techniques.

Specific lung expansion procedures and incentive spirometry are effective in preventing stiffness and decreased lung compliance. Through techniques that include low-flow, high-volume inspirations, expansion of the lung periphery is achieved. These techniques are especially useful in conditions such as localized atelectasis, pneumonia, pulmonary condensation and other pulmonary conditions of restrictive origin (9).

4.2.1. Distal or middle intrathoracic airways: Slow inspiratory techniques
- Controlled Inspiratory Debit Exercises (CIDE): Consists of slow and deep inspirations at low flow and high volume. It is performed in lateral decubitus with the area to be treated in supralateral position (non-dependent), while the physical therapist provides support from behind. Inspiratory volume is increased to total lung capacity (TLC), followed by a 3 to 5 second tele-inspiratory apnea to promote collateral ventilation and airflow to the peripheral air spaces (9).

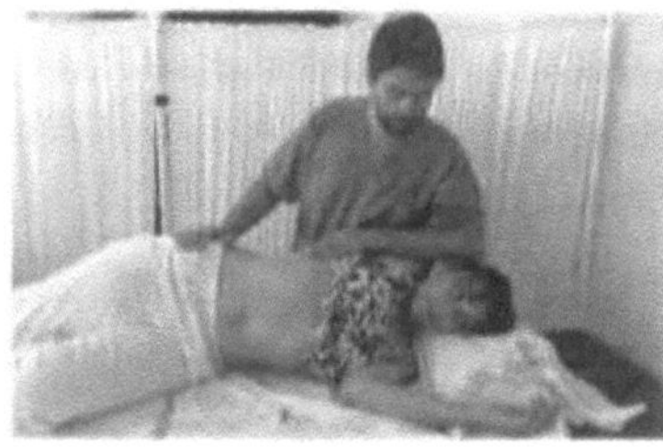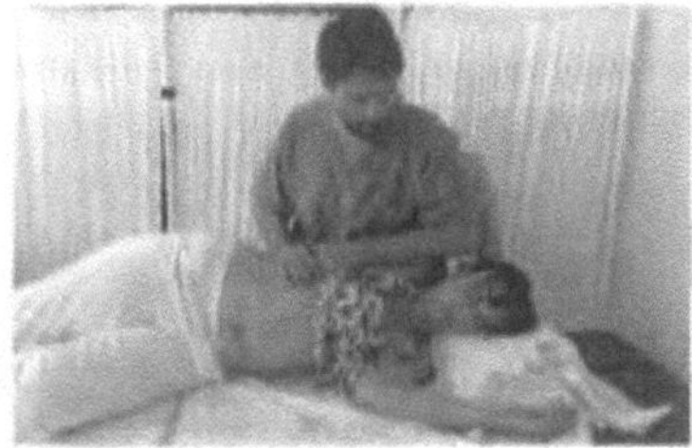

Figure 29. EDIC in inspiration (left figure) and EDIC in expiration (right figure) (9).

- Incentive Spirometry: Volume (Voldyne or Coach)®, Debit (Triflow)®: This technique is based on feedback, allowing the visualization of the volume of inspired air (volume) or the flow generated by the patient (debit). It must be ensured that the patient can use the device correctly and understand the instructions to avoid counterproductive effects. In addition to volume recovery, this technique mobilizes secretions from the deep lung into the middle airway. It is contraindicated in cases of inspiratory fatigue and untreated pneumothorax (9).
- Manual hyperinflation technique through a resuscitation bag (Air stacking): A resuscitation bag connected to the patient's mouth or to a tracheotomy is used to perform lung insufflation exercises. A pressure of 20 to 30 cm H2O is applied, synchronized with the patient's inhalations, followed by an apnea of 3 to 5 seconds. It is often accompanied by pressure on the abdomen or thorax to increase expiratory flows and reinforce ineffective coughing. This technique, which retains the maximum volume of air provided, may be useful in neurological patients with glottis control to facilitate expectoration (9).

4.3. Ventilatory techniques.

4.3.1. Proper use of the diaphragm

Diaphragmatic breathing is essential to reduce oxygen consumption and respiratory rate, resulting in greater respiratory efficiency and lower energy expenditure. The patient should focus on the diaphragm muscle and tidal volume, performing inhalations through the nose and exhalations through the mouth.

The position of the patient is crucial for the reeducation of the diaphragm dynamics. In the supine position, the diaphragm will be in the cranial position. In the supine position, the maximum displacement of the diaphragm occurs in the posterior region, whereas, in the prone position, maximum diaphragm re-education is achieved in the anterior region of the muscle. In lateral decubitus, it is on the support side of the diaphragm, on the underside of the side. In the seated or standing position, the diaphragm is in a low position due to gravity and the weight of the viscera, facilitating inspiration and hindering expiration. In this position, the diaphragm is in a caudal position, with greater expansion during expiration. On the contrary, in the supine or prone positions, expiration is facilitated and inspiration is hindered due to the position of the viscera, with a predominant expansion during inspiration. In the lateral decubitus position, we find a mixed expansion of the diaphragm. In the lower zone of the lateral side, the expansion is inspiratory (facilitating expiration and hindering inspiration), while, in the upper zone of the lateral side, the expansion is expiratory (facilitating inspiration and hindering expiration).

4.3.2. Targeted ventilation technique

The technique of targeted ventilation, described by Giménez in 1968, refers to respiratory awareness with the aim of modifying the ventilatory mode and automating the patient's abdomino-diaphragmatic breathing, either at rest or during exercise. This type of breathing helps to correct paradoxical movements and ventilatory asynchronisms, as well as to improve the sensation of shortness of breath. The methodology to obtain a new ventilatory rhythm is detailed below (23).

- PHASE I (1-2 weeks): Breathing awareness
    - At this stage, basic notions of respiratory anatomy and physiopathology are taught.
    - We work on the unblocking and harmonic use of the diaphragm.
    - Ventilatory asynergies are corrected.
    - The goal is to achieve a respiratory rate of 5-10 breaths per minute, adapted to each patient.
- PHASE II (longer, until the objectives are reached): Practice of targeted ventilation.
    - In this phase, the aim is to automate the new ventilatory rhythm.
    - Guided ventilation is practiced in various postures (supine, prone, lateral decubitus, seated, standing).

- Exercises of rib and shoulder girdle mobility are performed, as well as strengthening of the abdominal girdle, always in coordination with breathing.
  - The goal is to achieve a respiratory rate of 10-18 breaths per minute.
- PHASE III: Control of the new ventilatory rhythm
  - In this phase, control of the new respiratory rhythm is sought during activities of daily living (ADL).
  - Breathing rhythm control is practiced during exercise, avoiding associating breathing with walking. Monitoring by pulse oximeter is recommended.

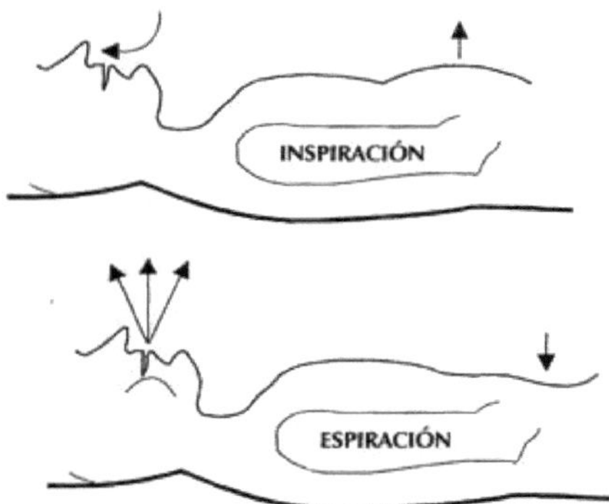

Figure 30. The initial exercise of the directed ventilation technique involves a deep, nasal inspiration, during which the abdomen expands forward. On exhalation, which is maximal, prolonged and performed against pursed lips, the abdomen contracts inward (23).

4.3.3. Abdomino-diaphragmatic directed ventilation technique:

This technique is based on diaphragmatic breathing to ventilate the lung bases. It consists of progressive deep inspirations, followed by an apnea of 3-5 seconds to favor the increase of collateral ventilation, and finally total exhalations with the lips clamped. By activating the diaphragm, the phrenic center descends and the viscera move outwards. It is performed with low frequency ventilation and high tidal volume (23).

4.3.4. Rib directed ventilation technique

This technique involves costal breathing, which mobilizes the different areas of the thorax, such as the upper ribs, the lower ribs, the right or left hemithorax, or a general mobilization of the entire thoracic area. Inspiration can be accompanied by raising the upper extremities and exhalation by lowering them to facilitate global thoracic mobilization. Costal ventilation is performed with slow and deep inspirations, followed by a 3-5 second apnea to promote collateral ventilation, and then a relaxed exhalation. It is used to improve ventilation in the middle and upper lungs (23).

- Upper or lower costal mobilization: The patient is placed in various positions and performs a tidal volume increase by directing the breath with manual stimulation to the upper ribs if mobilization of the upper costal area is intended, or by blocking the lower costal area if mobility of that hemithorax is to be hindered, and vice versa for lower costal mobilization.
- Mobilization of the left hemithorax or right hemithorax: The patient is placed in right lateral decubitus to mobilize the left hemithorax, and in left lateral decubitus to mobilize the right hemithorax.

4.3.5. Expiration with pursed lips

This technique consists of inhalations through the nose and slow exhalations with the lips in a whistling position. Pursed-lip ventilation helps to avoid premature airway closure and allows better lung emptying. The main objective of this technique is to reduce bronchial collapse, which leads to an increase in tidal volume and a decrease in respiratory rate, thus contributing to better gas exchange. This technique is indicated in several respiratory conditions, such as bronchospasm, cystic fibrosis, bronchitis, bronchiectasis, among others. It is especially useful in patients with chronic obstructive pulmonary disease (COPD), being the technique of choice in this case. It can be accompanied by facilitating positions to improve its effectiveness, such as the trident position (leaning forward with the elbows resting on the knees), leaning on a table, and even placing the head on the table to rest. These postures can help to optimize the pursed-lip exhalation process (23).

4.4. Instrumental devices.
4.4.1. Cough Assist®:

The Cough Assist® is a mechanical insufflation-exsufflation generator that reproduces the cough mechanism. During insufflation (produced by positive pressure), lung volume is increased, followed by exufflation (produced by negative pressure), which aims to evacuate bronchial secretions. This device is used in patients with amyotrophic lateral sclerosis, muscular dystrophy or other conditions involving respiratory muscle dysfunction in the muscles involved in coughing. It is also used in patients with respiratory infection and difficulty mobilizing secretions, with a peak cough flow of less than 270 l/min (4).

Contraindications for this device include emphysematous bullae, pneumothorax, hemoptysis, airway instability, recent barotrauma and hemodynamic instability. Pressure should be set between +-40 and +-50 cmH20, with an inspiratory time of 2-3 seconds and an expiratory time of 3-4 seconds. Air exit through the opening of the glottis will be favored (4).

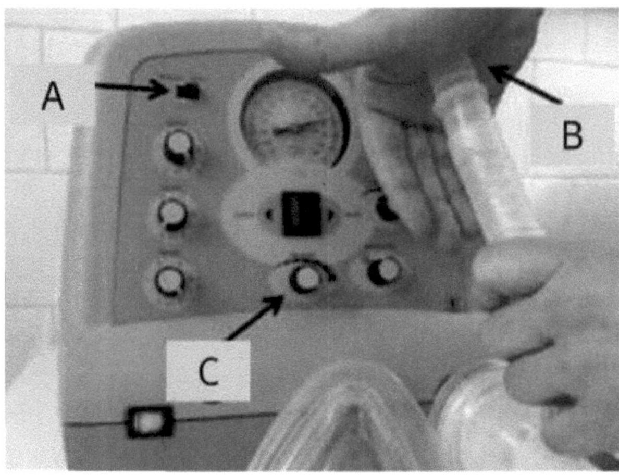

Figure 31. In automatic mode (A), we obstruct the tubing (B) and adjust the pressure (C) until it reaches the optimum treatment pressure (4).

4.4.2. Vibration Vests® (Vest®)

These external devices apply exogenous oscillation-compression vibrations at high frequency, compressing the rib cage and increasing transthoracic pressure. This generates micro-accelerations of expiratory flow that facilitate the elimination of bronchial secretions and reduce their viscoelasticity. Absolute contraindications include hemodynamic instability, hemoptysis and recent or unstable injuries, while relative contraindications include pneumothorax, emphysema, rib fractures, among others (4).

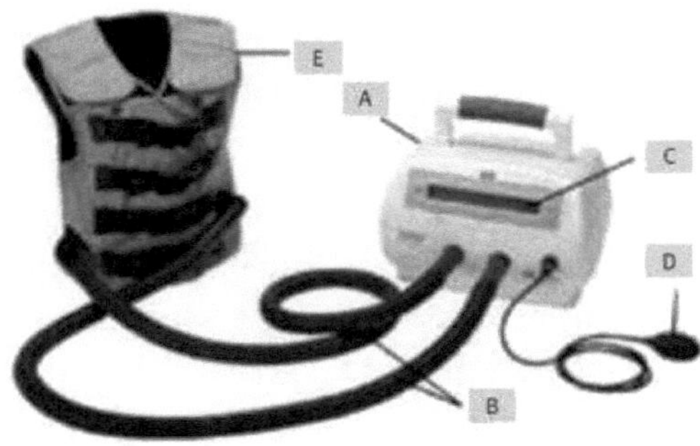

Figure 32. Pulsatile generator for high frequency chest wall compression (Vest®) (4).

4.4.3. Percussionaire

Percussionaire® is an intrapulmonary percussive ventilation technique that delivers high frequency, high flow, low pressure percussions to recruit collapsed alveoli or mobilize bronchial secretions in distal airways. It can be applied in acute or chronic cases of various respiratory pathologies, regardless of the patient's age and autonomy. Contraindications include undrained pneumothorax, hemoptysis and recent or unstable injuries. Recommended dosages vary according to the patient's condition and type of respiratory pathology. In patients with obstructive diseases, a working pressure of 1-2 bars is recommended, while in patients with restrictive diseases, a working pressure of 2-4 bars is suggested (9).

4.4.4. WBS devices

Positive expiratory pressure (PEP) devices offer resistance to airflow during expiration, which increases the duration of this phase and favors the opening of collateral ventilation and recruitment of collapsed alveolar regions. There are oscillating and non-oscillating devices. Examples include Flutter®, Acapella®, and Therapep®. Oscillating PEPs provide endogenous vibration, which helps modify the rheology of secretions and facilitates their expulsion. In the postoperative period following lung surgery, positive expiratory pressure during expiration (PEP) is intended to re-expand lung tissue. Oscillating devices are indicated in case of loss of bronchial wall stability. Contraindications include untreated pneumothorax, hemoptysis, sinusitis, otitis and facial surgery (4).

- Oscillating WBS devices (4):
  - Flutter®: The Flutter® is a "pipe" shaped device that includes a stainless steel ball in an enclosed space over a conical expiratory valve. When the user exhales through the device, the airflow pushes the steel ball, which bounces inside the valve, creating interruptions in the airflow and generating intermittent positive airway pressure (5-19 cmH2O). This produces oscillations in airflow between 6 and 26 Hz.
    - Patient position: seated. The inclination of the device can be adjusted to increase or decrease the resistance, which affects the positive pressure generated.
    - Patient instructions: breathe in slowly through the nose (or with the mouth open around the mouthpiece), take an inspiratory pause of 2-3 seconds and then perform an active exhalation through the device, keeping the cheeks rigid.
    - Exercise recommendation: combine 5-10 normal exhalations through the device with 1-2 forced exhalations outside the device (such as EFT or coughing) for 3-4 repetitions. The duration of the session can be 10-20 minutes.
  - Acapella®: Similar to the Flutter®, the Acapella® contains a counterweight plate with a magnet that covers an expiratory valve.

Exhalation through the device displaces the plate intermittently, creating oscillations in airflow and generating positive airway pressure. Unlike the Flutter®, the Acapella® has a gear to adjust the expiratory resistance and can be used at any angle or position. The exercise procedure is the same as described for the Flutter®.

- RC-Cornet®: The RC-Cornet® is a "horn" shaped device containing a rubber hose connected to a rotating mouthpiece. Exhalation through the device causes the mouthpiece to rotate, producing intermittent twists in the hose and generating oscillations in the airflow. Treatment with the RC-Cornet® is similar to Acapella® and a minimum treatment time of 10-20 minutes is recommended.

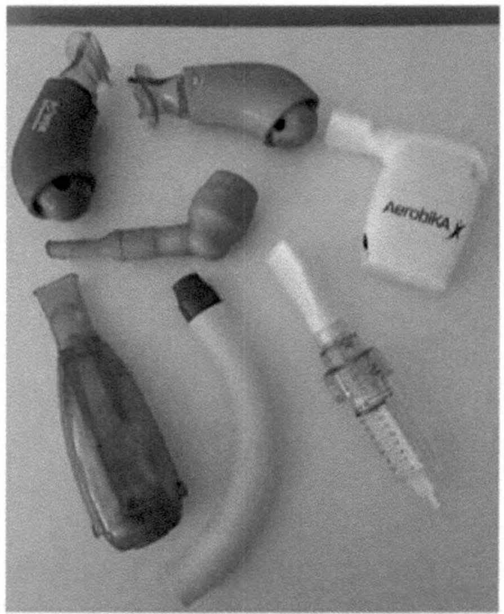

Figure 33. Oscillating WBS devices (4).

4.4.5. Respiratory muscle training devices

These devices, such as the Threshold® and Powerbreathe® threshold opening valve, are used to strengthen the respiratory musculature. Threshold® allows airflow to enter only after reaching a certain pressure, while Powerbreathe® is a specific training device for the respiratory muscles (9).

4.5. Other respiratory procedures.

4.5.1. Aerosol therapy

Aerosol therapy is a form of treatment that consists of delivering liquid or solid particles in a gas through a nebulizer or inhaler. This therapeutic approach makes it possible to administer substances or drugs by air, such as bronchodilators, corticosteroids, antibiotics and mucolytics, in order to achieve high therapeutic concentrations in the areas to be treated and to fluidize bronchial secretions. The action of the active principle is fast and local, and requires lower doses than other routes of administration, resulting in few side effects (9).

Nebulizers convert liquids into aerosol for deposition in the respiratory tract and therapeutic action. There are several types of nebulizers (23).

- Ultrasonic type: These nebulizers use the vibration of a piezoelectric crystal to fragment the liquid solution and produce aerosol. They are less common and are mainly used to nebulize water or saline.
- Jet type: Nebulizers of this type generate aerosol by means of a gas flow, which can be generated by an electric compressor or a gas compressor such as oxygen or air. They are suitable for nebulizing a wide variety of drugs.
- Vibrating mesh nebulizers: These nebulizers create aerosol by passing liquid through holes contained in a mesh. They are highly effective, achieving greater pulmonary deposition and lower drug loss compared to jet type nebulizers.

On the other hand, inhalers, such as pressurized inhalers (MDI) and dry powder inhalers (DPI), are devices used to generate aerosols of solid particles. The types of inhalers used for the treatment of the respiratory patient are (9):

- Pressurized or MDI (Metered Dose Inhalers): These inhalers are portable devices containing a plastic applicator with a cap.

Therapeutic particles are released at high velocity from a mouthpiece that is applied directly into the mouth or attached to a spacer chamber, such as a face mask. They are recommended for young children or elderly people with difficulty coordinating inhalation, as it is not necessary to synchronize inspiration with inhaler activation.

- Dry powder or DPI (Dry Powder Inhalers): These inhalers contain the medication in dry powder form. Each type of inhaler has specific instructions for use. They require minimal inspiratory flow by the patient, so in case of a crisis with inspiratory flow limitation, the use of an MDI inhaler is recommended.

Depending on the size and shape of the inhaled particles, they can be deposited in the respiratory system through three main mechanisms (9):

- By impaction: This mechanism occurs when aerosols are deposited on a surface due to a change of direction in the gas flow. The impinging particles are generally the larger ones, with a size greater than 5-6 µm. This process occurs mainly in the bifurcations of the upper airway, due to the high flows and turbulence present in this area.
- By sedimentation: In this mechanism, aerosols are deposited in the airways by the effect of gravity. The particles that are deposited are less than 6 µm and greater than 2 µm in size. This process occurs mainly in the lower airway and increases proportionally with apnea.
- By diffusion: particles in an aerosol move erratically through the airways due to Brownian motion. These particles are smaller, ranging in size from 3-2 µm to 1-0.5 µm mean aerodynamic diameter (dmda). Particles smaller than this size are expelled to the outside during expiration.

The inhalation technique is fundamental to ensure the efficacy of the treatment. Here is the correct sequence to facilitate drug deposition in the airway (9):

- Maximum and slow exhalation: The patient should perform a slow, full exhalation to empty the lungs of residual air and create space for inhalation of the medication.

- Deep inhalation: After exhalation, the patient should perform a deep and slow inspiration. It is important that the inhalation is gradual and continuous. Halfway through the inspiration is when the inhaler should be triggered to release the medication.
- Pause (apnea): Once the patient has inhaled the medication, he/she should pause briefly (apnea) for 3-5 seconds in adults and 2-3 seconds in children. This pause allows the drug to be distributed and deposited in the airways more effectively.
- Slow exhalation: Finally, the patient should exhale slowly, allowing the drug to settle in the airways and be absorbed properly.

Regarding the order of medication administration and physiotherapy treatment, it is recommended to follow this protocol (9):

- Hypertonic saline or bronchodilator treatment: It is administered first to open the airways and facilitate the elimination of secretions.
- Respiratory physiotherapy: After the bronchodilator, respiratory physiotherapy is performed to mobilize and eliminate accumulated secretions in the lungs.
- Antibiotic: If necessary, antibiotic is administered after respiratory physiotherapy to treat the underlying respiratory infection.
- By following this order, treatment efficacy is maximized and optimal improvement in the patient's respiratory function is ensured.

4.5.2. Oxygen therapy

Oxygen therapy is a therapeutic modality that increases the amount of oxygen breathed to improve oxygenation of vital organs, thus prolonging life and improving the quality of life in patients with respiratory failure. The decision to use oxygen therapy is based on an accurate measurement of blood oxygen levels by arterial blood gasometry. It is important to understand that oxygen therapy does not relieve the sensation of dyspnea, but rather addresses the objective lack of oxygen in the body. There are different devices to administer oxygen, which must be adapted to the specific needs of each patient and his or her disease. There are two broad categories of devices: low-flow systems and high-flow systems. Typical oxygen doses vary between 1 and 3 liters per minute (23).

- Low-flow systems: These devices provide a flow of oxygen that is less than the patient's inspiratory demand, meaning that the patient also inhales room air in addition to the supplemental oxygen. Examples of low-flow systems include nasal cannulas and nasal masks.
- High-flow systems: These devices deliver a flow of oxygen that is equal to or greater than the patient's inspiratory demand, ensuring that the patient inhales a constant concentration of oxygen regardless of his or her breathing pattern. Examples of high-flow systems include face masks and high-flow nasal cannulae.

The choice of the appropriate device depends on several factors, such as the severity of respiratory failure, the patient's specific oxygenation needs and comfort (23).

- Low-flow systems in oxygen therapy involve the patient inhaling ambient air mixed with the supplied oxygen. The final inspired oxygen concentration (FiO2) cannot be accurately determined and varies according to several factors, including the device used, the prescribed oxygen flow rate, and the patient's respiratory characteristics (23).

  - Nasal Goggles (NG): These are flexible plastic tubes with two protrusions that are inserted into the patient's nostrils. They are comfortable and allow the patient to talk, eat, etc. This makes them popular for home oxygen therapy. However, at high flows they can cause irritation or nasal bleeding if humidification is not used. The FiO2 obtained can vary between 26-40%, but no specific oxygen concentration can be guaranteed.
  - Simple Mask: A flexible plastic mask that fits over the patient's face, with a connection for oxygen delivery. The space between the mask and the patient's face acts as an enlargement of the natural reservoir, allowing higher blood oxygen concentrations to be achieved than with nasal goggles, in the range of approximately 0.4-0.6. However, as with nasal goggles, the final FiO2 depends on the patient's breathing pattern and no specific

concentration can be guaranteed. It is important to avoid too low oxygen flows to avoid carbon dioxide rebreathing and to prevent pressure ulcers on the nasal septum and ears. In addition, too high flows may cause irritation and dryness of the eyes due to oxygen leaking from the sides and top of the mask.

- Mask with Reservoir: This mask is similar to the simple mask, but has an attached plastic reservoir that increases the volume of air available to the patient. The reservoir bag can hold between 600-1000 ml of air. This bag allows to increase the natural reservoir and to maintain a more stable oxygen concentration in the mask. It has two one-way valves on the sides of the mask to allow the exhaled air to exit and prevent carbon dioxide rebreathing and the entry of ambient air. In addition, there is a third one-way valve between the mask and the reservoir bag that allows the passage of oxygen into the mask, but prevents the passage of exhaled air into the bag. This device is capable of providing oxygen concentrations very close to 100%, provided that certain requirements are met, such as correct adaptation to the patient's face, keeping the reservoir bag full at all times and ensuring that the three one-way valves are correctly positioned. This type of mask is indicated for patients requiring tighter control of FiO_2, such as in cases of carbon monoxide poisoning, heart failure, acute pulmonary edema, among others. In addition, it allows treating hypoxemia and symptoms until the underlying cause improves, avoiding the need for intubation.

- High-flow systems: High-flow systems are devices that have the ability to deliver oxygen at higher concentrations than ambient air, ensuring a specific inspired oxygen fraction (FiO_2), regardless of the patient's breathing pattern (23):

  - Venturi Mask (Air Entrapment Mask or Ventimask): This system uses the Bernoulli effect to deliver oxygen at specific concentrations regardless of the patient's breathing pattern. Oxygen enters the device through a small-bore orifice, which causes ambient air to be drawn in through the side orifices. This mixture of oxygen and room air increases the available airflow in the mask. The FiO2 obtained will depend on the oxygen flow and the opening of the side windows of the mask. This device allows FiO2 values between 24% and 50% to be achieved. It is important to provide humidification when oxygen flows greater than 4 liters per minute are used. In addition, it is crucial to relate the FiO2 delivered to the oxygen flow in liters per minute according to each manufacturer's specifications.

- High-flow nasal goggles are devices designed to deliver oxygen at a high flow rate through the patient's nostrils. These goggles have larger caliber nasal cannulas than conventional nasal goggles, allowing flows of up to 60 liters per minute (l/min) to be achieved. The main benefit of high-flow nasal goggles lies in their ability to provide high FiO2 and ensure sufficient flow that can match or exceed the patient's inspiratory flow. In addition, these systems are often equipped with a humidification and heat circuit that helps improve patient tolerance and prevent side effects associated with high airflows, such as nasal dryness or mucosal irritation. Importantly, the beneficial effect of these devices is not only limited to increasing FiO2, but the constant high airflow can also have positive effects on the patient, such as decreasing dead space by creating an oxygen reservoir in the patient's airway and the effect of continuous positive airway pressure during expiration, which can improve alveolar ventilation and tissue oxygenation.

- Oxygen delivery is accomplished by various oxygen generating devices or sources. These devices include (23):
  - Oxygen concentrator: This device extracts oxygen from the ambient air and separates it from nitrogen, which increases the concentration of oxygen available to the patient. The air we normally breathe contains approximately 21% oxygen, and the concentrator increases this proportion. It is especially useful for home oxygen therapy.
  - Oxygen cylinder: This is a cylindrical device usually made of steel. It consists of three main parts: a pressure gauge, a tap and a flow meter flow selector. Oxygen cylinders contain oxygen compressed

at high pressure, which is released through the flow regulated by the flowmeter. This type of device is commonly used in hospitals and medical environments.

- Liquid oxygen tank or nurse: This device stores oxygen in liquid form at very low temperature, which allows the oxygen to remain in a liquid state. When needed, the liquid oxygen is transformed into a gas when delivered to the patient at room temperature. From these liquid oxygen tanks, portable backpacks can be filled, allowing mobile and flexible oxygen administration.

Each of these devices has its own advantages and is used depending on the specific needs of the patient, location and clinical conditions.

5. <u>RESPIRATORY REHABILITATION TRAINING PROGRAM</u>

Respiratory rehabilitation (RR), as defined by the American Thoracic Society and the European Respiratory Society, is a comprehensive intervention based on a thorough patient assessment, followed by personalized therapies that include, among other things, muscle training, education and lifestyle changes. It aims to improve both the physical and emotional condition of people with chronic respiratory disease and promote adherence to long-term healthy behaviors. RR has proven to be one of the most effective non-pharmacological treatments for patients with chronic respiratory diseases, such as COPD. However, there is growing evidence of its effectiveness in other respiratory and non-respiratory conditions, such as asthma, cystic fibrosis, bronchiectasis, interstitial lung diseases, pulmonary hypertension, neuromuscular diseases and rib cage deformities. In addition, it has been observed that it can reduce complications in lung resection surgeries and in the pre- and post-transplantation period (28).

It is important to bear in mind that respiratory rehabilitation programs do not improve pulmonary function tests. This implies setting realistic goals so as not to generate unrealistic expectations in both patients and health professionals.

- The main objectives of the RR are (28):
  - Improve exercise tolerance
  - Reduce dyspnea
  - Increase physical and social participation
  - Improve autonomy in daily activities
  - Reducing the use of healthcare resources
  - Promote lifestyle changes and improve quality of life.

- The sequence of a respiratory rehabilitation program generally follows the following steps (28):

- Patient selection: It will depend on the characteristics of the program and the patient's clinical situation.
- Initial evaluation: Each potential candidate should be evaluated clinically, radiologically and functionally by his or her treating physician to confirm the diagnosis and determine the appropriate pharmacological treatment.
- Determine realistic objectives and goals: Once the patient has been selected and his or her health condition has been assessed, realistic objectives and goals for the rehabilitation program should be established.
- Define the components of the program: Based on the established objectives and the patient's individual needs, a program will be designed that may include muscle training, education about the disease, changes in lifestyle habits, among other components.
- Outcome evaluation: During and at the end of the program, outcomes will be evaluated to determine the effectiveness of the treatment and make adjustments if necessary.

Patient selection will depend on the criteria of the rehabilitation program and the specific clinical situation of each individual. The initial evaluation will include tests such as assessment of inhalation technique, exercise tolerance by laboratory and field tests, respiratory muscle function, assessment of dyspnea and health-related quality of life (28).

- Components of respiratory rehabilitation programs include (28):
  - Lower extremity aerobic exercise: This is the fundamental component and is performed using cycloergometers, treadmills or other modalities such as walking or swimming. It is recommended two to five times per week for 30 to 45 minutes per session, with high workloads and a minimum duration of 8 weeks.
  - Upper extremity aerobic exercise: Improves arm strength and endurance and is performed using arm ergometers, elastic bands or small weights.
  - Strength training: Increases strength and peripheral muscle mass. High intensity, low repetition exercise is recommended, one to three sets of 8 to 12 repetitions, two to three times per week.

- Respiratory muscle training: Improves respiratory muscle strength and endurance, especially in COPD patients. It is recommended to perform it once to twice a day, for five days a week, using threshold pressure devices.
- Education: Focuses on knowledge of the disease, self-care, prevention and treatment of exacerbations, as well as energy-saving techniques.
- Psychosocial support: Evaluates and treats anxiety and depression concomitant with chronic respiratory disease, using specific questionnaires and referring to specialists as needed. Respiratory rehabilitation has been shown to be effective in reducing these symptoms, although more studies are needed to confirm this.

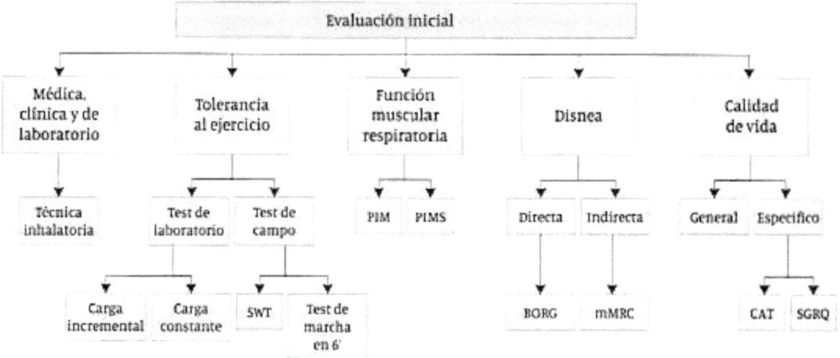

Figure 34. Algorithm for initial patient assessment for entry into the respiratory rehabilitation program (28).

5.1. Ventilation and costal expansion exercises.

The purpose of these exercises is to improve lung elasticity and capacity, as well as to prevent the accumulation of mucus plugs common in cystic fibrosis. It is advisable to perform these exercises prior to the bronchial hygiene techniques mentioned above. It is crucial that air reaches all areas of the lung to facilitate mucus clearance through the drainage techniques mentioned above (31).

- Targeted ventilation exercises can be performed in various positions to impact different lung areas (lying on the back, side, sitting and standing). They focus on three types of respirations (31):
  - Abdomino-diaphragmatic: Place one hand on the abdomen and one on the chest. Breathe in deeply through the nose, directing the air toward the hand on the abdomen without moving the chest. Then exhale gently and slowly to deflate the abdomen.
  - Lower rib cage: Place your hands on the ribs on both sides of the chest. Breathe in deeply through your nose, feeling the opening of the lower ribs. Then exhale gently and slowly to close the ribs.
  - Upper thoracic: Place one hand on the chest. Breathe in deeply through your nose, directing the air into that area of your chest. Then, exhale gently and slowly to deflate the chest.

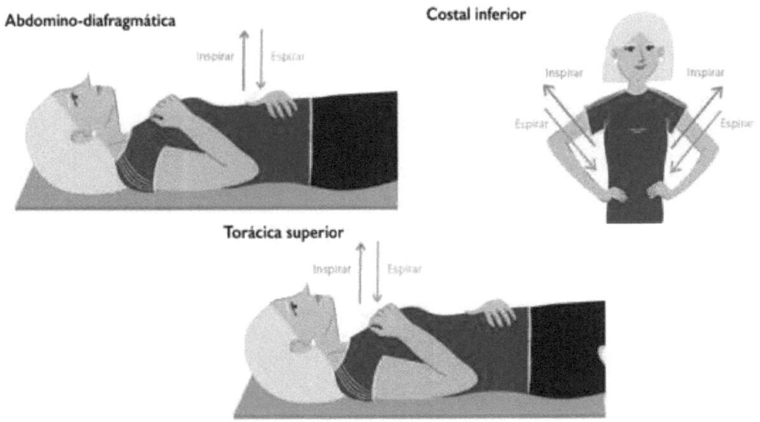

Figure 35. Representation of targeted ventilation exercises (31).

- Rib expansion: Thoracic expansion exercises can be combined with arm movements and performed in different positions to achieve a more complete expansion in specific areas of the lungs. Several examples are described below (31):
  - Exercise I: Sitting with the back supported, inhale through the nose opening the arms in a cross and exhale closing the arms and hugging the thorax. It can also be done by lifting the arms forward or to the sides.

- Controlled Inspiratory Debit Exercise (CIDE): Lying on your side with your leg and arm straight. The exercise consists of expanding the upper lung by inhaling deeply through the nose while raising the arm to expand the ribs. The air is held for 3 to 5 seconds, then exhaled slowly while lowering the arm. You can increase the rib opening by placing yourself on a cushion.

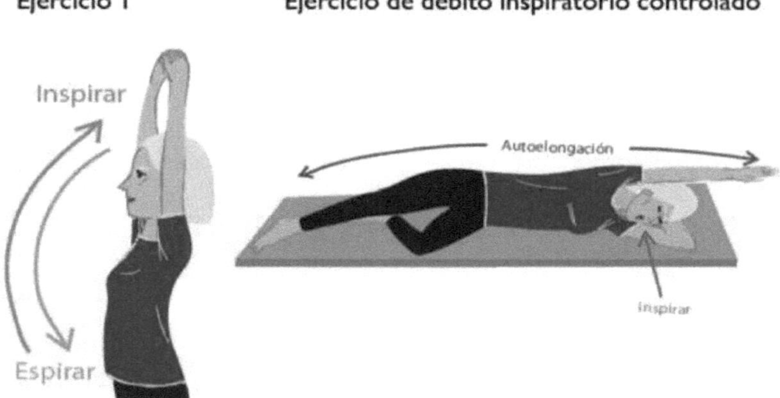

Figure 36. Representation of exercises in rib expansion (31).

5.2. Recommendations for home physical exercise.

Home physical exercise is essential in the treatment of respiratory diseases, as it not only maintains physical condition in an optimal state, but also significantly improves the prognosis of the disease. Among the most relevant benefits at the pulmonary level are the slowing of lung function deterioration, improved ventilation and bronchial mucus clearance, as well as the reduction of air trapping in the lungs and the increase in lung capacity. From the musculoskeletal point of view, exercise increases muscular strength and endurance, favoring exercise tolerance, and improves bone mass, which prevents the onset of osteopenia and osteoporosis. Finally, from a psychological point of view, exercise provides a feeling of well-being, improves neuronal connections, learning, memory and brain plasticity, which helps to reduce states of depression.

In short, physical exercise at home produces a great improvement in the quality of life (31).

Recommended weekly dose: Children and adolescents should engage in at least 60 minutes of moderate-intensity physical activity on all or most days of the week, or vigorous-intensity physical activity 3 days a week. Adults should engage in at least 150 minutes of moderate-intensity physical activity per week, or 75 minutes of vigorous-intensity physical activity, including a combination of both (31).

- Recommended type of physical exercise (31):
  - Aerobic exercise: Includes activities that involve the cardiovascular system, such as walking, running, swimming or cycling.
  - Strength and muscular endurance exercises: These focus on strengthening muscles through the use of weights, elastic bands or body resistance exercises, such as push-ups or squats.
  - Flexibility exercises: They help to improve the elasticity and range of motion of the joints, such as static or dynamic stretching.
  - The combination of these three types of exercises has proven to be effective in improving respiratory function, increasing muscle mass and improving quality of life in people with respiratory pathology.

- General recommendations (31):
  - During an exacerbation of the disease, it is recommended to reduce the duration of the exercise session and increase the weekly frequency.
  - It is important to remember that physical exercise can cause coughing, but this should not be a reason to stop unless it is excessively uncomfortable or painful.
  - The training load should be personalized according to the individual characteristics of each person, including the number of repetitions, the weight used, the speed of execution and the duration of the exercise. It is recommended to follow the indications of the physiotherapist.

- In patients with severe airway obstruction, a cardiopulmonary stress test is recommended before starting a physical exercise program.

- Special precautions (31):
  - It is important to monitor oxygen saturation using a pulse oximeter during and after exercise. If saturation drops below 90%, it is recommended to stop exercise and rest until it returns to normal values.
  - It is also crucial to monitor the intensity of the workout. If you experience shortness of breath, excessive fatigue or inability to carry on a conversation during exercise, it is recommended to stop the exercise and rest or reduce the intensity.

- Home exercise guidelines (31):
  - Warm-up: About 10 minutes are dedicated to exercises involving all joints to activate the cardiovascular system and prepare the muscles and joints for the effort.

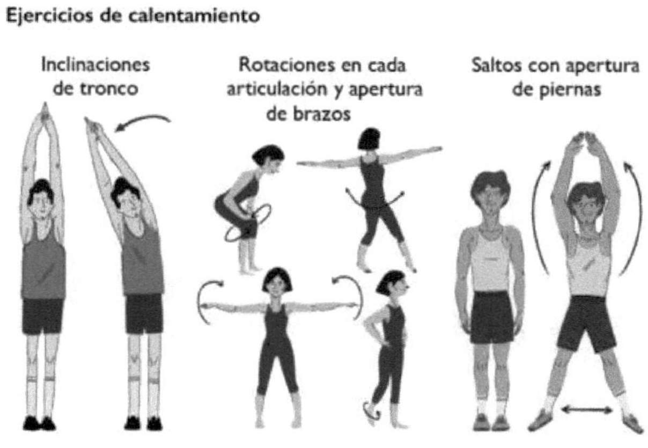

Figure 37. Recommended warm-up exercises (31).

- Aerobic exercise: Combine aerobic exercise with strength exercises. It is important to calculate and control the intensity of the exercise. The intensity is controlled in two ways:

- Heart rate: Calculate the maximum theoretical heart rate and do not exceed 80% of this rate if the pulmonary involvement is mild or moderate, or 70% if it is severe.
- Perceived exertion scale: Maintain perceived exertion between 3 and 8 on a scale of 10, depending on the level of training.

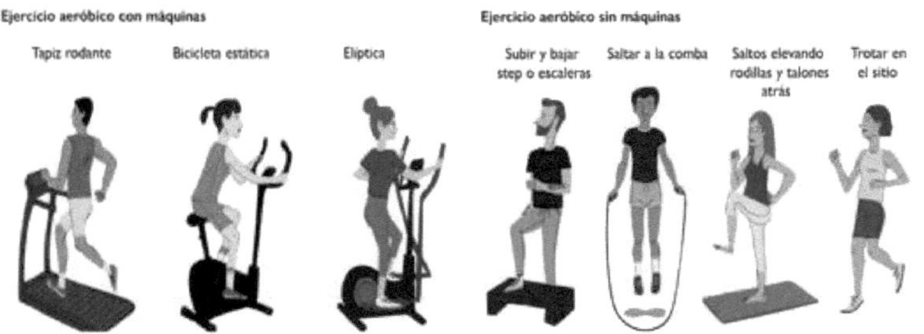

Figure 38. Aerobic exercise recommendation (31).

- Muscle strength and endurance exercises: Strengthen all muscle groups with exercises using dumbbells, water bottles, elastic bands, among others. Perform 2-3 sets of 10-12 repetitions for each exercise.

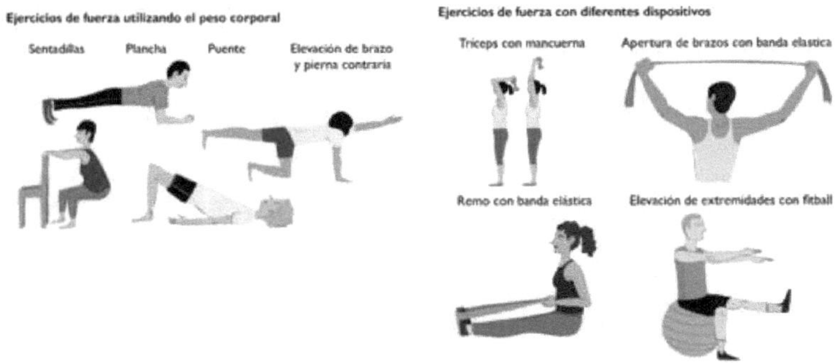

Figure 39. Recommended muscle strengthening exercises (31).

- Stretching: Perform stretches of each muscle group for about 30 seconds to improve flexibility and prevent injury.

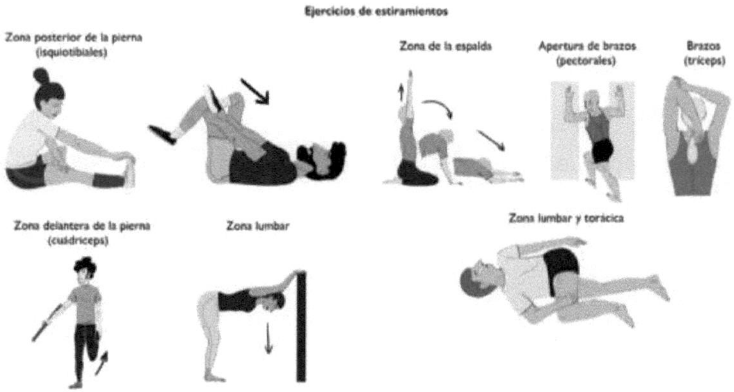

Figure 40. Exercise recommendations for stretching (31).

- Pilates and therapeutic yoga: These disciplines can benefit people with cystic fibrosis, improving lung capacity, oxygenation and strengthening the respiratory and abdominal muscles. It is important to learn these techniques with a specialized instructor.
- Remember to adapt the exercise according to the level of physical condition and follow the recommendations of the physiotherapist or physician.
- The following is a model recommendation for people with cystic fibrosis according to pulmonary involvement (31).

Pulmonary involvement	Mild or moderate (FEV1≥40%).	Severe (LVEF <40%)
Recommended activities	- Cycling - Walk - Hiking - Aerobic exercises - Career - Rowing - Tennis - Swimming - Strength training - Climbing - Skating	- Stationary bike - Walk - Strengthening exercises - Gymnastics - Daily activities

	• Trampoline	
Type of training	Interval and continuous	Interval
Frequency	3-5 times a week	5 times a week
Duration	30-45 minutes	20-30 minutes
Intensity	60-80% Fc max	50-70% Fc max.

Table 11. Recommendation of a physical activity program for people with cystic fibrosis (31).

5.3. Pelvic floor exercises.

Stress urinary incontinence is common and occurs when the pelvic floor muscles are weakened. During activities such as coughing, intra-abdominal pressure increases, which compresses the bladder and can lead to urine leakage. To combat this problem, pelvic floor contraction exercises, also known as Kegel exercises, can be performed (31).

- To perform the slow Kegel exercise in a lying position, follow these steps (31):
  - Lie on your back with the soles of your feet flat on the floor and your knees bent.
  - Raise the pelvis upward, forming a bridge with the body.
  - Breathe in deeply and, as you exhale, contract your pelvic floor muscles.
  - Imagine that you are closing and lifting the orifices (urethra, vagina and anus) into the pelvis, as if they were an elevator, for 4-5 seconds.
  - After the contraction, relax the muscles and lie back down completely, resting for at least 10 seconds to allow the muscles to recover.
  - Repeat this exercise slowly 15 times.
  - Over time, you can gradually increase the contraction time for better results.

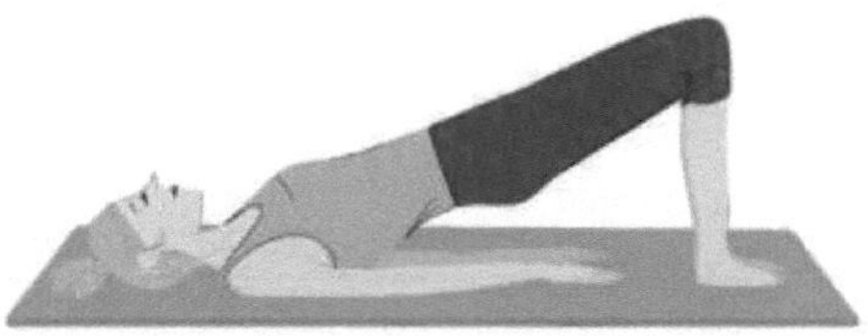

Figure 41. Representation of slow Kegel exercise in lying position.

- Rapid Kegel exercise to integrate perineal contraction into daily life (31):
  - Quickly contract your pelvic muscles while contracting your abdominals, as if you were hiding your navel.
  - At the same time, lengthen the trunk as if you were being lifted by a string from the head.
  - Hold the contraction for 1 second and then relax for 5 seconds.
  - Repeat this cycle 10 times.
  - It is advisable to perform this exercise several times throughout the day, especially during times of exertion, such as when lifting weights or performing intense breathing exercises.
  - As a complement to these exercises, hypopressive abdominal gymnastics, under the supervision of a specialized physiotherapist, can have beneficial effects on the pelvic floor.
- Knack technique during coughing or straining: The "Knack technique" involves voluntarily contracting the pelvic floor before coughing or straining to reduce pressure on and protect the pelvic floor, which can help prevent or reduce urine leakage. It is important to avoid flexing the trunk too much when coughing so as not to increase pressure on the pelvic floor. Over time, this technique will become automatic, and the pelvic floor will contract automatically in response to straining (31).

6. <u>RESPIRATORY PHYSIOTHERAPY IN THE CRITICALLY ILL PATIENT</u>

5.4. Physiotherapy in mechanically ventilated patients.

Mechanical ventilation (MV) is a method that uses external mechanical means to control and assist ventilation in patients with acute respiratory failure or decompensation of chronic pulmonary pathologies. This process is divided into several phases (38):

- Trigger: This phase marks the transition from expiration to a new inspiration. It is the moment when the ventilatory cycle starts.
- Inspiratory time: This is the period during which inspiration takes place. The duration of this phase depends on the assigned control parameters, such as pressure or volume, and is limited by a predefined maximum value.
- Cycling: The process of transition from the inspiratory phase to the expiratory phase in each ventilatory cycle. This can occur in three ways:
    - Volume-based: When the programmed volume is reached.
    - Time-based: When the inspiratory time predefined by the operator is reached.
    - Flow-based: A flow cutoff point is established, usually at 25% of peak flow. When the flow reaches this value, the ventilator considers that the patient is ending the inspiratory phase and the expiratory phase begins.
- Exhalation: This is the phase between one inspiratory cycle and another, where exhalation of the inspired air occurs. Generally, this phase is passive, and the duration of expiration will depend on several factors, such as respiratory rate and inspiratory time, as well as the ventilatory mode used.

There are several modes of mechanical ventilation that can be classified as complete (the patient does not participate or remains passive) and partial (the patient collaborates during respiration) (38):

- Controlled Mechanical Ventilation (CMV): In this mode, all the characteristics of the respiratory cycle are completely determined by the ventilator, and the patient cannot intervene. It is a completely passive mode of ventilation.
- Assisted Controlled Mechanical Ventilation: In this modality, ventilation is controlled by the ventilator, but the patient can initiate respirations and receive additional breaths if his inspiratory effort reaches a predetermined level.
- Synchronized Intermittent Mandatory Ventilation (SIMV): This system allows the patient to intersperse spontaneous breaths between ventilatory cycles controlled by the ventilator.
- Spontaneous Ventilation: In this mode, the patient breathes by himself. It can be subdivided into:
- Pressure Support (PSV): Each inspiratory effort of the patient is assisted by the ventilator up to a programmed inspiratory pressure limit (38):
    - Continuous Positive Airway Pressure (CPAP): The ventilator maintains a predetermined level of positive airway pressure throughout the respiratory cycle to keep the airway open.
    - Biphasic Positive Airway Pressure (BIPAP): Two pressure levels, one expiratory and one inspiratory, are applied to reduce the work of breathing and promote alveolar ventilation.
    - Pure Spontaneous Ventilation: The patient ventilates spontaneously through the ventilator circuit without receiving positive airway pressure. This method is used to assess whether the patient can be weaned from mechanical ventilation.

Consequences of mechanical ventilation may include (38):

- Reversal of the ventilatory cycle: In mechanical ventilation, air enters the airway producing a positive pressure instead of a negative intrathoracic pressure as in physiological respiration. Exhalation remains passive, but there may be an uneven distribution of ventilation between the lungs.
- Loss of upper airway filter function: When ventilating through an endotracheal tube or tracheostomy, the natural defenses of the upper airway are cut off from airflow.

- Alteration of mucociliary transport: Mechanical ventilation may interfere with the normal movement of mucus along the airways.
- Increased risk of infections: Due to loss of filter function and impaired mucociliary transport, patients on mechanical ventilation are at increased risk of respiratory infections.
- Respiratory muscle atrophy: Inactivity of the respiratory muscles during prolonged mechanical ventilation can lead to their atrophy.
- Complications of intubation: These include ulcers, airway strictures or fistulas, vocal cord problems and trauma.
- Pulmonary complications: such as pneumothorax and interstitial emphysema.
- ICU-associated muscle weakness (IUAD): A decrease in strength and generalized muscle atrophy, which may affect the peripheral and respiratory musculature.
- Hemodynamic effects: These include a decrease in cardiac output, decreased venous return and difficulty filling the left ventricle.

It is essential to minimize the patient's dependency time on mechanical ventilation systems due to these potential complications.

Mechanical ventilation can be invasive or noninvasive (38):

- Invasive mechanical ventilation (IMV):
  - It is performed through an endotracheal route by intubation (oral or nasal) or tracheotomy.
  - The objectives include providing effective ventilation without escape, avoiding inhalation of nasopharyngeal secretions or gastric fluid, and preventing airway obstruction.
  - A disadvantage is the need to find substitutes for natural functions such as air filtration, humidification and heating.
- Non-invasive mechanical ventilation (NIV):
  - Refers to any ventilatory support modality that does not require the insertion of an endotracheal line.
  - It has advantages over IMV, such as avoiding complications associated with intubation (infections, trauma, vocal cord problems) and not requiring sedation, since the patient can actively participate.

- Although NIV also has cardiovascular effects due to the increase in intrathoracic pressure, as well as the risk of alveolar overdistension.
- It is commonly used in exacerbations of chronic lung diseases such as COPD, but also has other applications with obvious benefits.
- The choice of interface (nasal, full face or helmet) is crucial to the success of the technique, and must be adapted to the patient's needs and comfort.

ICU-acquired muscle weakness is a crucial factor for physiotherapists to be aware of, as it can affect between 25% and 100% of patients on mechanical ventilation, even for short periods of time on the machine. To diagnose and evaluate this condition, several methods are available, including muscle biopsy, electromyogram, assessment of skeletal muscle strength using the Medical Research Council Scale (MRCss), and inspiratory muscle strength using maximal inspiratory pressure (Pmax) (39).

The simplest and most widely accepted tool to diagnose this weakness is the Medical Research Council Score (MRCss) scale. This scale assesses the strength of different muscle groups using specific movements, as outlined in the Hamilton (1992) and Hermans (2016) protocol. It is crucial to perform a comprehensive assessment of muscle strength using the MRC scale to determine the presence of ICU-acquired weakness. One begins by assessing muscle strength to obtain an MRC score of 3 and then continues with the test to achieve an MRC score of 4 or MRC score of 2, depending on the result obtained. This scale has a total score of 60, and a total MRC score of less than 48 indicates ICU-acquired weakness. In addition to the evaluation of muscle strength, in critically ill patients it is essential to assess a series of clinical and ventilatory parameters, such as blood gases, oxygen saturation, signs and symptoms, pulmonary auscultation, radiographs, cardiac function, symmetry in body temperature and perimeters, among others (39).

MEDICAL RESEARCH COUNCIL SCORE (MRCss)

VALUE	INTERPRETATION	MOVEMENT TO BE EXPLORED IN EACH LIMB
0	Absence of movement	• Abd arm
1	Visible contraction without movement	• Forearm flexion
		• Wrist extension
2	Motion without gravity	• Hip flexion
3	Full movement against gravity	• Knee extension
4	Complete movement against resistance	• Dorsi Flexion of the foot.
5	Normal force	

Table 12. Scale for presence of acquired weakness in the ICU. Medical Research Council Score (MRCss) (39).

5.5.   Role of the physiotherapist in critically ill patients.

Physiotherapy techniques play a crucial role in the management of patients undergoing mechanical ventilation, with the aim of maintaining adequate bronchial hygiene, improving respiratory function and facilitating the weaning process from ventilation. Here is a summary of the main techniques used (40):

- Hydration: It is essential to fluidize bronchial secretions and facilitate their mobilization. Humidifiers or aerosols can be used for this purpose.
- Drainage techniques: These include autogenous expiratory flow therapy (AFE), postural drainage, cough learning, expectorations, thoracic percussions, vibrations (such as mechanical insufflation-exsufflation and high frequency oscillations) and aspiration of secretions.
- Hyperinsufflations: Deep inspirations are performed with an incentive or manually with an ambu or ventilator.
- Postural changes: These are performed every 30 minutes to stimulate ventilation in different lung areas.
- Early mobilization: Activates the cardiovascular system and can facilitate recovery.
- Diaphragmatic exercises: They help to improve lung ventilation and respiratory function.

To facilitate weaning from mechanical ventilation, the following actions are carried out (38):

- Training of the respiratory musculature.
- Cough assessment to ensure sufficient capacity (greater than 65 l/min).
- Provide information and support to the patient.
- Proper postural care.
- Early mobilization of the extremities and cervical spine, adapted according to the patient's level of consciousness.
- Use of sedation rating scales, such as the Ramsay scale, Rich-mond Agitation-Sedation Sedation Scale (RASS), the Sedation-Agitation Scale (SAS), and the Motor Activity Assessment Scale (MAAS), among others.

It is important to take into account the safety criteria for physiotherapy treatment in the ICU, such as patient stability for at least 12-24 hours and the absence of "red flags" indicating risk. We consider the following parameters to be red flags for mobilization in the ICU (38):

- Temperature above 38.5° or below 36°.
- HR less than 40 bpm or greater than 130 bpm
- TAS less than 60 mmHg or greater than 180 mmHg
- TAD less than 50 mmHg or greater than 110 mmHg
- Saturation less than 90%
- Respiratory rate greater than 40 resp/min
- Inotropics, vasopressors in the 2 hours prior to the treatment.
- Level of consciousness RASS: -4,-5, 3, 4
- Uncontrolled pain
- FiO2 greater than or equal to 0.6
- PEEP greater than or equal to 10 cmH2O

RASS SCALE		
-5	Non-awakenable	DOES NOT respond to voice or physical stimuli
-4	Deep sedation	Moves or opens eyes to physical stimulation, not to the voice

-3	Moderate sedation	Eye opening movements to the voice, does not direct gaze.
-2	Light sedation	Awakens to voice, maintains eye contact less than 10 seconds
-1	Drowsiness	Not fully alert, stays awake for more than 10 seconds
0	Awake and at ease	
1	Restless	Anxious, no disorderly movements, no violent behavior
2	Shaken	Moves haphazardly, struggles with ventilator
3	Very hectic	Aggressive, attempts are made to pull out tubes and catheters.
4	Combative	Violent, represents an immediate danger to personnel

Table 13. Scale for sedation assessment. Rass scale (38).

During the weaning phase, the objective is to withdraw mechanical ventilation in a safe manner adapted to the patient's needs, aiming for promptness but maintaining safety. The criteria for weaning include parameters such as respiratory mechanics, respiratory muscle strength, ventilatory demand, ventilatory reserve, oxygenation, patient status according to the Glasgow scale and the T-tube spontaneous ventilation tolerance test (38).

If the period of mechanical ventilation has been brief, a rapid disconnection can be considered, switching to spontaneous ventilation mode or even totally disconnecting the patient from the ventilator, provided the patient's condition allows it. In prolonged cases, a progressive disconnection should be performed, passing through various phases. The patient may switch to an intermittent ventilation mode, where he or she breathes spontaneously between ventilatory cycles controlled by the ventilator. Positive end-expiratory pressure is also added to keep the alveoli expanded. Techniques should be employed to raise the patient's awareness of diaphragmatic breathing, increase the volumes of air mobilized, and use biofeedback to monitor respiratory rate and tidal volume. In addition, bronchial clearance techniques are continued (38).

Subsequently, we switch to a spontaneous ventilation mode, where the patient breathes on his or her own, but continues to be monitored. Correct diaphragmatic breathing is insisted upon and bronchial clearance techniques are maintained. Periods of mechanical ventilation in spontaneous mode alternate with periods where the patient is released from the ventilator, providing additional oxygen as needed (38).

The weaning phase ends when the patient is deintubated and weaned from mechanical ventilation. If necessary, noninvasive ventilation by face mask can be used. During this stage, respiratory physiotherapy techniques are continued to improve bronchial clearance and ventilatory mechanics, as well as mobilizations to avoid muscle atrophy. Finally, in cases where necessary, unscheduled extubation may be performed due to problems such as inadequate sedation or poor fixation of the endotracheal tube (38).

5.6.   Respiratory physiotherapy in the postoperative period.

Airway patency is crucial to ensure adequate airflow in the tracheobronchial tree and to facilitate alveolocapillary exchanges. Several factors can contribute to bronchial obstruction by accumulation of secretions, such as postoperative pain, inability to produce an effective cough, reduced lung volumes, increased work of the respiratory muscles, and infections that affect the consistency of secretions. To mobilize pulmonary secretions and direct them into the trachea, various strategies are employed (40):

- Verify patency and clean secretions adhered to the nasogastric tube.
- Humidify the tracheobronchial tree by means of aerosols.
- Dislodge secretions using manual vibrations or instruments.
- To favor secretion drainage by increasing expiratory flow, avoiding abrupt exhalation to prevent early alveolar collapse.
- Facilitate expulsion of secretions with directed coughing or expiratory throat clearing, taking care to avoid excessive increases in intra-abdominal pressure and unproductive coughing spells.

- Use positive expiratory pressure ventilation techniques, such as lip-clamped expiration, incentive spirometry and specific mechanical devices.

In case of intubation, excess secretions will be removed by suctioning, with the help of the physiotherapist to mobilize them by manual pressure on the thorax and abdomen during expiration. Combating altered respiratory mechanics and ventilatory disturbances is essential to improve pulmonary function after surgery. The aim is to increase tidal volume, reduce respiratory frequency and correct imbalances in the distribution of ventilation to prevent atelectasis, which is present in most operated patients (40).

To address these goals and stimulate diaphragmatic activity, various techniques of targeted ventilation (DV) and diaphragm reeducation are applied (40).

- Global ventilation at low frequency and high volume, either spontaneously or with the aid of incentive spirometry.
- Gentle active exhalation to bring the diaphragm to a high position and increase its travel.
- Localized targeted ventilation, focusing initially on increasing tidal volume in a general way and then concentrating on specific areas of hypoventilation. Diaphragmatic breathing can be performed in a semi-sitting position with manual support from the physiotherapist, accompanied by tele-inspiratory apnea.
- Localized costal breathing, where the patient directs inspiration towards the operated or specific area to be worked on, with manual stimulation by the therapist to guide the respiratory movements and avoid complications.
- Periodic changes of position to prevent hypoventilation in declined areas, avoiding the Trendelemburg position.
- Passive, assisted and active kinesitherapy to maintain joint mobility.

These techniques aim to restore normal respiratory mechanics and improve pulmonary ventilation after surgery.

7. <u>PEDIATRIC RESPIRATORY PHYSIOTHERAPY.</u>

In infants, totally passive techniques will be applied, while in children aged 18-24 months, their participation will be encouraged through play during therapies.

- Upper airway cleaning: nasal lavage (31).

To perform upper airway clearance, a syringe and hypertonic saline solution (~2.3% NaCl) should be used. These nasal cleansing techniques help remove secretions and facilitate proper breathing in infants and young children.

- Nasal lavage in infants without head/trunk control:
  - Place the child on its back.
  - Gently hold the chin or head with one hand.
  - Administer the serum (1-2.5 ml per nostril) slowly and without pressure in each nostril to avoid choking.
  - Then, perform the chin-up maneuver or cover the mouth so that the child performs forced inhalations through the nose, dragging the phlegm towards the throat, where he/she will cough or swallow.
- Nasal lavage in infants with head/trunk control:
  - Sit the child on the therapist's legs with the back resting on the abdomen.
  - Tilt the child forward to drain secretions from the nostrils.
  - Administer the saline (2-5 ml per nostril) with a little more force so that it comes out through the other nostril.
  - Clean the posterior area by leaning backwards and administer the serum slowly (1-3 ml in both nostrils).
  - Cover the child's mouth so that he/she breathes in strongly through the nose, drawing the phlegm into the throat, where he/she will cough or swallow.

Focus on older children and collaborators:

For older children and collaborators, we can ask them to participate by asking them to inhale strongly through their nose, using motivating phrases such as: "What does it smell like?", "I think it smells like...", "Let's see who can inhale faster and stronger", "You have to inhale strongly like an elephant's trunk", etc.

- Bronchial secretion drainage (41):

There are two types of techniques: those that mobilize or collect secretions from more distal areas (distal) to those closer to the bronchial tree (proximal), and techniques to evacuate secretions found at the proximal level. It is recommended to perform both techniques in each session, always starting with those directed to the distal areas and then the evacuatory ones. It is suggested to take advantage of the benefits provided by laughter or crying, since they help the drainage of secretions due to the increased flow and the vibration they generate.

- Techniques for collecting bronchial secretions distally in infants and young children:
  - Prolonged slow exhalation: With the child lying on the back and with a slight trunk elevation of 20-30°, one hand is placed on the chest and the other on the abdomen. Slow pressure is applied to lengthen the exhalation and drag the phlegm from distal to proximal. The maneuver is repeated as many times as necessary to evacuate the secretions.

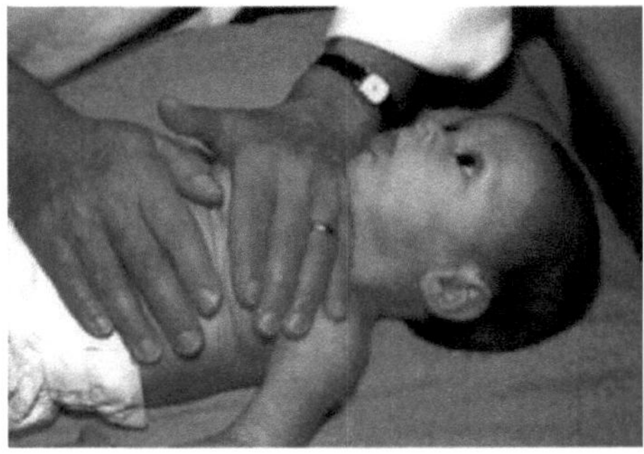

Figure 42. Representation of prolonged slow expiration in infants (ELPr) (41).

- Prolonged open-glottis slow expiration (OLSE): The application modalities of OLSE can be active-passive or active. In the active-passive technique, the patient is positioned in lateral decubitus and performs slow exhalations from Functional Residual Capacity (FRC) to Residual Volume (RV). The physical therapist can provide assistance by standing behind the patient and applying infralateral abdominal pressure with one hand, while exerting counter-pressure at the level of the supralateral rib cage with the other hand. This pressure, directed towards the contralateral shoulder, promotes the most complete possible infralateral lung deflation. The patient can also perform ELTGOL autonomously, although periodic monitoring of the performance is required due to the tendency of patients not to follow the technique correctly (41).

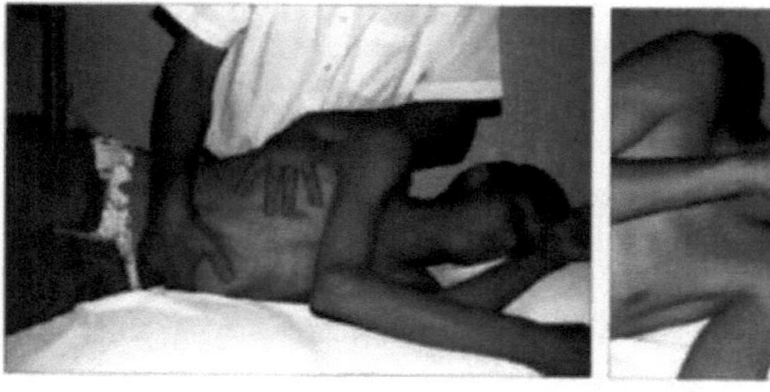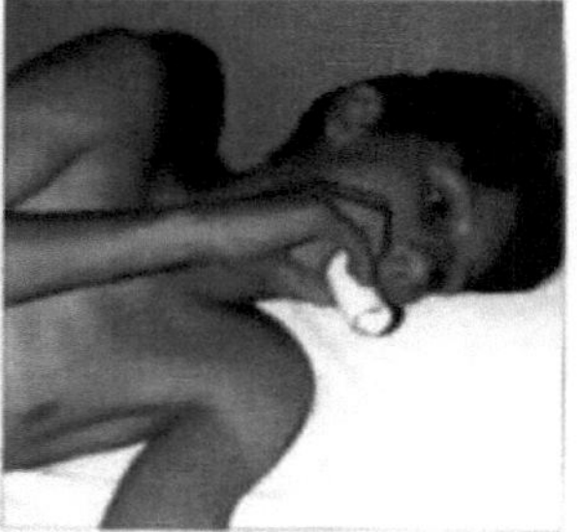

Figure 43. Prolonged slow expiration with open glottis (ETGOL) (41).

- Autogenic Drainage: The site and mode of action of Autogenic Drainage (AD) are closely linked to the general mechanisms of slow exhalations. AD shares similarities with Therapeutic Slow Sclerosis of the Great Laryngeal Oscillations (TLGSOL). DA has been validated to have superior effects to forced expiratory techniques, especially in the middle airways. Proponents of the method promote a ventilatory mode that is based on fractional expirations, starting from fractional volumes of Total Lung Capacity (TLC), with the aim of obtaining higher bronchial debits than those achieved during forced expirations. They use criteria such as pulmonary function tests and the number of expectorations collected to validate the efficacy of the method. Although there are no scintigraphy data to accurately place the effects of DA on the tracheobronchial tree, it is presumed to generate better small airway debits based on the shape of the debit/volume curve. Proponents of DA suggest that, through control of expiratory debit, patients may develop a kind of habituation. This would mean that the patient can influence the cough reflex by lowering the threshold of bronchial irritability, which would reduce the need to cough during the bronchial clearance process, which is highly beneficial in chronic diseases (41).

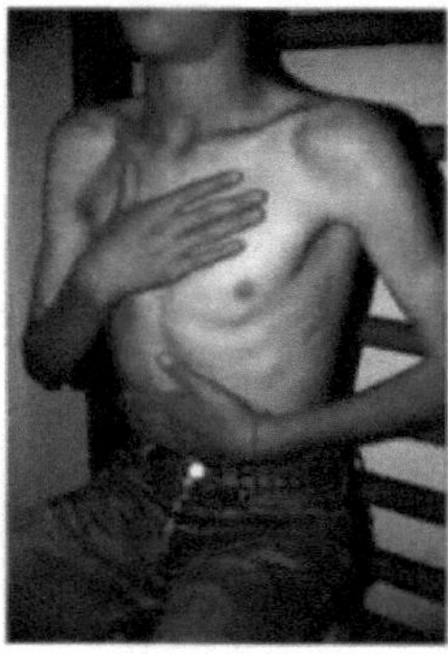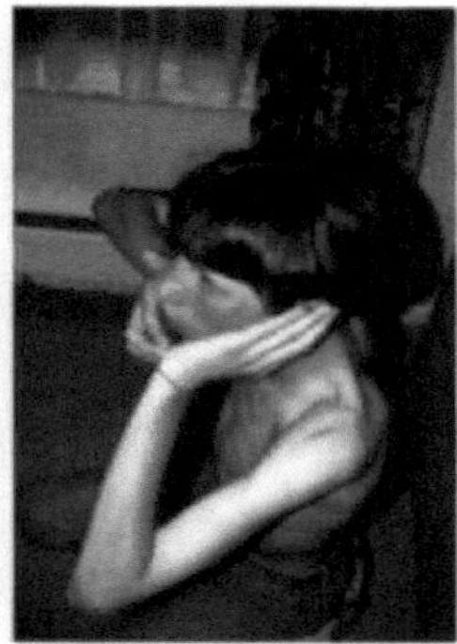

Figure 44. Autogenous drainage performed by the patient himself (41).

For physiotherapist-assisted autogenous drainage, it is recommended that an elastic strap be placed under the armpits, covering the child's chest and abdomen to provide consistency to the rib cage and improve the function of the respiratory musculature. The hands are placed around the child's chest with both thumbs facing each other at the level of the sternum. A light pressure is applied towards the child's navel to achieve a slow exhalation and promote emptying, trying to slightly block inspiration. The maneuver is repeated as necessary to evacuate the secretions (31).

- Techniques to evacuate secretions at the proximal level in infants and young children:
  - Increased expiratory flow: With the child lying down or sitting, rapid and short thoracic and abdominal pressures are performed to mobilize secretions in the proximal airways and evacuate them into the throat.
  - Provoked cough: To induce cough in a controlled manner, we will place the child semi-incorporated and, after a deep inhalation, we will apply a quick and gentle pressure on the middle of the neck above the sternum. This will activate the productive cough reflex. It is important not to repeat this technique several times to avoid irritating the area. It is recommended to use this technique only if, after performing the techniques to collect secretions at the distal level, the child does not cough involuntarily.

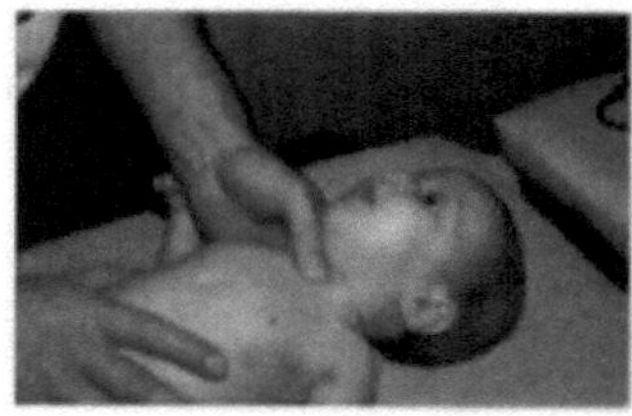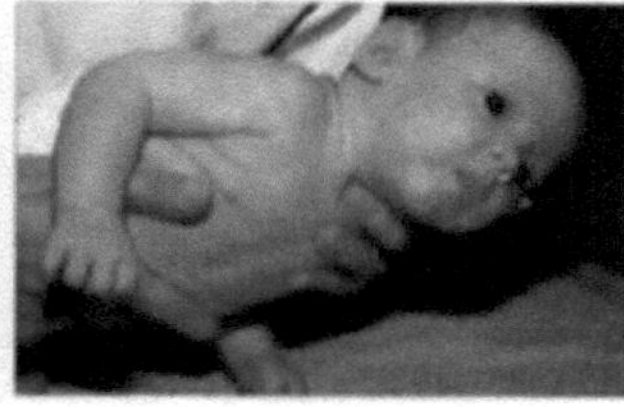

Figure 45. Representation of provoked cough in infants (41).

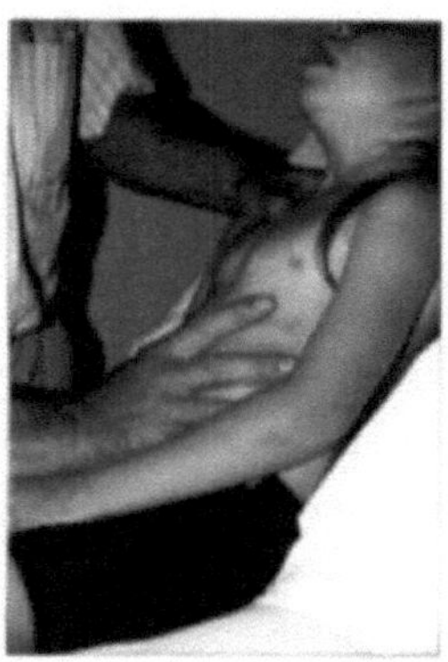

Figure 46. Directed cough in children (41).

- Expiratory tracheal pumping (ETP) emerges as an innovative and effective technique for the management of severe accumulations of secretions in the proximal airways, especially in situations where the cough reflex is diminished or absent, as in certain neuromuscular diseases in infants and young children. This technique, developed from empirical observation and clinical intuition, has proven effective in mobilizing tracheobronchial secretions and expelling them into the oropharynx, thus relieving acute respiratory distress. BTE is based on a physical reference model that resembles the operation of a pump, where pressure exerted along the trachea by peristaltic movements of the thumb moves secretions from the proximal airways to the more distal airways. This approach requires a trachea with a high compliance, which makes it particularly suitable for young children with unconsolidated tracheal cartilages. The indications for BTE focus on situations of respiratory urgency caused by accumulation of secretions in the proximal airways, although its use should be limited to selected cases and under strict control of oxygen saturation. Importantly, this technique should be applied with caution and is contraindicated in cases of local pathology of the extrathoracic trachea. Although BTE represents a significant advance in the management of respiratory secretions, its validity and safety must continue to be studied and validated, especially through clinical observations and experimental studies in anatomical models. Ultimately, BTE offers a new perspective in the therapeutic arsenal of respiratory physiotherapy, with the potential to improve clinical outcomes and quality of life for patients with severe respiratory disorders (41).

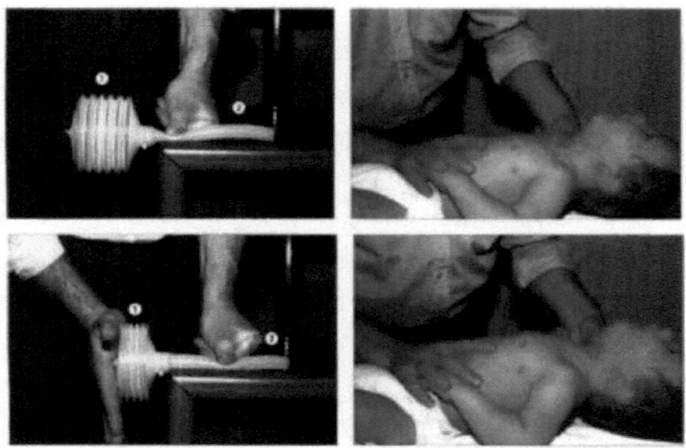

Figure 47. Expiratory tracheal pumping maneuver (BTE). (41).

- Games to promote drainage of secretions (31):

The games should involve expirations and inspirations adapted to the child's abilities, without neglecting the respiratory physiotherapy techniques previously described. Some activities that aid secretion drainage and thoracic expansion include:

- Making bubbles: With a straw in a glass or a pipe in the bathtub.
- Flow ball, blopens (airbrush markers), blowing ping-pong balls or polystyrene balls: Create circuits or play soccer by blowing.
- Singing songs, playing an instrument (harmonica, trumpet) or learning to whistle.
- Activities such as jumping on a trampoline or sitting on a fitball.

In the techniques for older children and adults to clear the upper airways, we will use a jar or a nasal irrigator with isotonic or hypertonic saline. We will perform a nasal lavage to drain secretions from the nostrils, tilt the head and apply the saline through the upper nostril until it comes out of the other nostril. Then, we will make strong and deep inspirations to mobilize the secretions towards the throat, where they can be coughed and expectorate. After nasal lavage, it is recommended to evacuate the excess secretions using the appropriate technique.

- Evacuation technique (31):

The nasal blowing evacuation technique may be less effective than others, but it is sometimes necessary to remove excess secretions from both nostrils. First, it is important to teach the child to blow through the nose. This can be accomplished by placing a light object, such as a polystyrene ball, on a table and encouraging the child to move it by blowing through the nose. You can also practice blowing through the nose with a straw into a glass of water.

Once the child has learned to blow through the nose, to evacuate nasal secretions correctly, follow these steps:

- Occlude a nostril with the finger.
- Blowing air forcibly through the nose, evacuating secretions from the free nostril.
- Repeat the process with the other nostril until the excess secretions are completely evacuated.
- Cautions: Never occlude both nostrils at the same time, as this may increase internal airway pressure and displace secretions into other passages, such as the ear canals. It is important to be careful when teaching this technique and to supervise the child to avoid injury or complications.

In conclusion, respiratory physiotherapy plays a fundamental role in the management and treatment of various respiratory conditions, both acute and chronic. Through a variety of techniques and approaches tailored to the individual needs of each patient, this discipline seeks to improve pulmonary ventilation, promote secretion clearance, optimize respiratory mechanics and improve overall lung function. From weaning from mechanical ventilation to the treatment of chronic respiratory diseases such as cystic fibrosis or asthma, respiratory physiotherapy addresses a wide range of conditions. Its holistic approach, combining manual techniques, breathing exercises, patient education and, in some cases, the use of assistive devices, aims to improve quality of life and reduce respiratory complications. Respiratory physiotherapy is an invaluable tool in respiratory care, working closely with other healthcare professionals to provide a comprehensive, multidisciplinary approach to the treatment and management of respiratory disease.

BIBLIOGRAPHIC REFERENCES

1. González, F., Méndez F., Vargas E., Benavides, J. (2009). Respiratory physiotherapy: general aspects. Revista Médica Clínica Las Condes, 20(6), 769-775.

2. Rodríguez, J. M. G., Candel, A. G. (2006). Respiratory physiotherapy and its practical applications. EdikaMed.

3. Pryor, J. A., Prasad, S. A. (2008). Physiotherapy for respiratory and cardiac problems: a guide to practice. Elsevier Spain.

4. Bañala, A., et al. (2013). Manual SEPAR de Procedimientos 27 Manual and instrumental techniques for bronchial secretion drainage in the adult patient. Barcelona: Respira-Fundación española del pulmón-SEPAR. ISBN: 978-84-941669-0-7.

5. Troosters, T., Langer, D., Vrijsen, B. (2016). Pulmonary rehabilitation and respiratory physiotherapy. European Respiratory Journal, 48(1).

6. Thomas, P., Bruton, A., Littlewood, C. (2010). Respiratory physiotherapy for chronic obstructive pulmonary disease. Cochrane Database of Systematic Reviews, (5).

7. West, J. (2022). Pulmonary pathophysiology: Fundamentals. Wolters Kluwer Publishing House. ISBN: 978-8418563836

8. Bott, J., et al. (2009). Guidelines for the physiotherapy management of the adult, medical, spontaneously breathing patient. Thorax. 64 Suppl 1:i1-i51.

9. Seco, J. (2021). Respiratory system: methods, clinical physiotherapy and conditions for physiotherapists. Panamericana. ISBN: 978-8491102038

10. Sebbagh, E. et al. (2012). Radiological anatomy of the thorax. Rev.chil. Enferm.respir, Vol.8, no.2. pp. 109-137. http://dx.doi.org/10.4067/S0717-73482012000200005

11. Moore, K. L., Dalley, A., Agur, A. (2018). Anatomy with clinical orientation. 8th edic Wolters Kluwer. ISBN: 978-8417033637

12. Atlas of anatomy. Version 2024.0.05 (Mobile application). Developer Visible Body. 2007. IOS or Android platform.

13. Koeppen, B., Stanton, B. (2018). Physiology. 7th Edic Elsevier. ISBN: 978-8491132585.

14. Cristancho, W. (2012). Respiratory physiology, the essentials in clinical practice. 3rd edition Editorial El Manual Moderno. ISBN: 978-958-9446-61-4.

15. García, H. F., Gutiérrez, S. E. (2015). Basic aspects of airway management: anatomy and physiology. Mexican Journal of Anesthesiology. Vol 38(2) pp: 98-107.

16. Guyton, Hall, J, E. (2016). Treatise on medical physiology. 13th Edition Elsevier. ISBN: 978-8491130246

17. Farias, G. (2004). Gasometry: Acid-base balance in the clinic. 2nd Edition Manual Moderno. ISBN: 9789707291423

18. Mejía, H., Mejía, M. (2012). Pulse oximetry. Journal of the Bolivian society of pediatrics. 51(2): 149-155. ISSN: 1024-0675

19. Cabrera, P., et al. (2005). Manual of respiratory diseases. 2nd edition International union against tuberculosis and respiratory diseases. ISBN: 2-914365-22-5.

20. García, F., Gómez, M.A. (2011). Functional respiratory exploration. Neumomadrid. ISBN: 978-84-8473-983-8.

21. Gutiérrez, M., et al. (2018). Spirometry: Manual of procedures. SERChile. Revista Chilena de Enfermedades Respiratorias. 34:171-88. ISSN 0717-7348

22. Marcelina, S., et al. (2021). Evaluation of lung capacity as a function of tidal volume in university students during the COVID-19 pandemic. Peruvian Journal of Health Sciences. 3(4): 256-60.

23. Cristancho, W. (2008). Fundamentals of Respiratory Physiotherapy and Mechanical Ventilation. 2nd edition Manual Moderno. ISBN: 978-958-9446-25-6

24. Puente, L., et al. (2002). SEPAR manual of procedures. Spanish Society of Pneumology and Thoracic Surgery. ISBN: 84-7989-152-1.

25. Baéz, R., et al. (2016). The exploration of the thorax: a guide to decipher its messages. Journal of the Faculty of Medicine of the UNAM. 59(6).

26. Arcas, M.A., et al. (2006). Respiratory physiotherapy. Editorial MAD. ISBN: 84-665-5384-3

27. Campignion, P. (2000). Respir-Actions: Muscle and joint chains G.D.S. Lencina verdu. ISBN: 9788460703129

28. Arancibia, F. (2020). Manual of respiratory diseases. Editorial Mediterraneo. ISBN: 978-956-220-428-6.

29. Burgos, F., et al. (2004). SEPAR manual of procedures module 4: Pulmonary function assessment procedures II. Spanish Society of Pneumology and Thoracic Surgery. ISBN: 84-921622-3-6

30. Conesa, E. (2019). Clinical evaluation of the response to respiratory physiotherapy in children diagnosed with acute bronchiolitis. International doctoral school. Catholic University of Murcia.

31. Camarero, P., et al (2020). Manual of respiratory physiotherapy for people with cystic fibrosis: Volume 1 respiratory physiotherapy and physical exercise recommendations. Spanish group of physiotherapy for cystic fibrosis. Madrid Association of Cystic Fibrosis. ISBN: 978-84-09-23996-2

32. Vilaró, J., Gimeno, E. (2016). Effectiveness of respiratory physiotherapy in asthma: respiratory techniques. Revista de Asma. 1(2) pag: 41-45.

33. Leon, J., et al. (2019). Chronic obstructive pulmonary disease. Junta de Andalucía: Consejería de Salud y Familias. ISBN 978-84-949160-7-6.

34. Herrero, M.V., García, A., Rositi, E., Villalba, D. (2023). Respiratory physiotherapy in adult subjects hospitalized for community-acquired pneumonia. Annals. 56(2): 109-116

35. Ruiz, M.E., Pareja, P., De la Sierra, M., García, M. (2011). Functional recovery after repeated pneumothorax: Respiratory physiotherapy treatment. Clinical case. Rehabilitation Service of the General University Hospital of Ciudad Real.

36. Martínez, C., Cols, M., Salcedo, A., Sardon, O., Asensio, O., Torrent, A. (2014). Respiratory treatments in neuromuscular disease. Annals of pediatrics. 81(4): 259.e1-259.e9.

37. Postiaux, G. (2016). Kinésithérapie et bruits respiratoires. De Boeck Publishing House. ISBN: 9782807303072

38. Ramos, L.A., et al. (2012). Fundamentals of mechanical ventilation. Barcelona: Marge Médica Books. ISBN: 9788415340508.

39. Hermans et al (2016) Protocol for assessing limb muscle strength in critically ill patients admitted to the ICU: the Medical Research Council Scale.

40. Update in respiratory rehabilitation (2023). Spanish Society for Cardio-Respiratory Rehabilitation (SORECAR). ISBN: 978-84-09-57716-3

41. Postiaux, G. (2000). Respiratory physiotherapy in the child. McGraw-Hill. ISBN: 84-486-0269-2

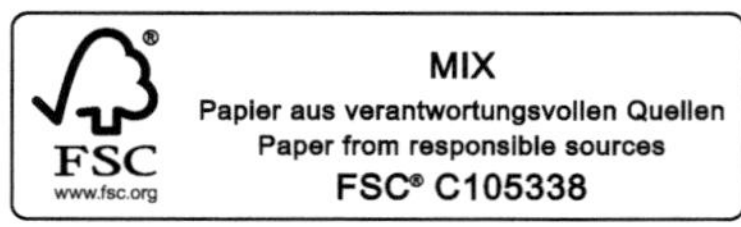

Printed by Books on Demand GmbH, Norderstedt / Germany